PSYKHE

ABOUT THE AUTHOR

Richard Carlton Crabtree is a Director of the Oakdale Well-being Group and has worked in mental health, at the forefront of the Department of Health's flagship 'Improving Access to Psychological Therapies' (IAPT) programme, for more than ten years, having led the expansion of IAPT into more than thirty regions around the UK. He has been a Director and Trustee of several charitable health, sporting and wellness organisations close to his home in Yorkshire, has written about mental health and psychological therapies for the *Independent* newspaper, and contributed to national forums shaping mental health policy. Prior to this Richard read Economics and Economic & Social History at the University of York and worked in the public sector with the Ministry of Defence.

@rdcc1000

PSYKHE

THE MENTAL HEALTH CRISIS AND HOW WE GOT HERE

R. D. C. CRABTREE

AMBERLEY

First published 2021

Amberley Publishing
The Hill, Stroud
Gloucestershire, GL5 4EP

www.amberley-books.com

Copyright © R. D. C. Crabtree, 2021

The right of R. D. C. Crabtree to be identified as the Author of this work has been asserted in accordance with the Copyright, Designs and Patents Act 1988.

ISBN 978 1 3981 0271 2 (hardback)
ISBN 978 1 3981 0272 9 (ebook)

British Library Cataloguing in Publication Data. A catalogue record for this book is available from the British Library.

1 2 3 4 5 6 7 8 9 10

Typesetting by SJmagic DESIGN SERVICES, India.
Printed in the UK.

CONTENTS

ACKNOWLEDGEMENTS

With heartfelt thanks to my friends and colleagues Lorian Rein, James Brandon, Scott Denison, Brendan Hill, Dr Esther Cohen-Tovee, Dr Caroline Falconer, Dr Leahan Garrett, Steven Ibbotson and Michael Rein for their insightful critiques of the early draft of this book. I am also particularly grateful to Connor and the whole team at Amberley Publishing for their enormous contribution to getting the work, and the word, out. Thanks too to Sarah-Jayne, Charles, Louis and especially to S. P. Crabtree for a lifetime of loving support. Finally a major thank you to Sir Norman Lamb for providing the foreword for *Psykhe*, and for his own long dedication to the cause of promoting good mental health.

FOREWORD

Most will have heard of the 'one in four' statistic for those who will experience mental illness. Mental health problems are often utterly debilitating, and, without effective support, can destroy people's lives. Most families are touched by mental ill health and ours is no exception.

During my eighteen years as a Member of Parliament, I was repeatedly confronted by the failures of our mental health system. So often people told me how they, or their loved ones, had been let down by the system. Long waiting times, high thresholds to even get accepted onto a waiting list, people still institutionalised, endemic use of force, regular use of compulsory detention. These are all features of a dysfunctional system which too often fails to respect people's human rights and which also fails to focus sufficiently on how we prevent mental ill health in the first place.

More positively, in those eighteen years, I did notice a shift in attitude not only in government but also in society.

When I became Minister for Care and Support in 2012 during the Coalition, I was committed to unpicking what I felt was historic discrimination built up over centuries and to help put mental health onto the map and onto the government's agenda. There was an institutional bias against it, reflecting the stigma of mental health in society. I championed parity of esteem – mental health being given the same priority as physical health – and helped introduce the first ever maximum waiting time standards for the treatment of mental ill health. We've still got such a long way to go, but there are lots of ways in which mental health is now ignored less than it was in the past. When Theresa May became prime minister, she singled out the lack of support available for people experiencing mental ill health as one of her seven 'burning injustices', showing, at the very least, a wider change in the recognition of the inequality suffered by those experiencing mental ill health. This was the first time that a prime minister in the UK had directly and publicly prioritised mental health. Yes, there is a gap between the rhetoric and the reality, but we should welcome this new focus. Then there have been public campaigns like 'Time to Change' to raise awareness and combat stigma. This has helped to encourage open conversations. The willingness of public figures, including young members of the royal family, to talk about their own personal experiences, perhaps makes it just a bit easier for a teenager to speak out and get help.

This excellent book tracks the wider changes in society, particularly in the last century, which have shaped experiences of and attitudes towards mental health. Richard Carlton Crabtree tackles the rise of social media and the impact that this has on our mental health, which is now a widespread topic of conversation. As Chair of the Science and Technology Select Committee in Parliament, I led an Inquiry looking into the impact of social media and screen-use on young people's health. Social media can be a force for good, helping to bring people together from across the world to share their creativity and passions, but it can also lead to people feeling more isolated and result in increased pressures around body image. It can facilitate cyberbullying. And then there has been one of the defining moments of this generation with the lockdown imposed by most countries during the Covid-19 crisis. The psychological fallout from this crisis is likely to be profound with lost jobs, financial distress, businesses built up through years of toil destroyed and loved ones lost.

In the following chapters, Richard charts all the extraordinary highs and lows, the leaps forward and the steps backwards, in society's attitudes towards mental ill health, from the Ancient Egyptians' supernatural explanations to the effects of wartime and the impact of the digital age. Whilst there remains a great deal of work still to be done, I believe that we are making real progress in addressing the institutional bias that has previously stopped mental health getting the attention it deserves – and, as Richard outlines, we all have our own role in changing things for the better.

Sir Norman Lamb
Chair of the South London and Maudsley
NHS Foundation Trust
Founder of Sir Norman Lamb
Mental Health & Well-being Fund
Minister of State for Care and Support 2012–15

THE BREATH OF LIFE – A PROLOGUE

Psykhe is the Greek goddess of the soul. To ancient Greeks the meaning of her name would have been taken as *'animating spirit'*, or the more poetic *'breath of life'*. Our most complete account of her story comes from Platonicus, written in the second century AD.[1] It describes how Venus, the goddess of love, becomes so jealous of Psykhe's beauty that she persuades Cupid to shoot one of his arrows into her as she sleeps, with the intention of causing Psykhe to fall in love with a beast Venus planned to have planted in her bedroom.

Instead, it is Cupid who unwittingly pricks himself with his own arrow and falls in love with Psykhe, and when the frustrated Venus curses the union so that they cannot marry, Cupid responds by refusing to shoot any more enchanted arrows until Venus relents and lifts her curse. Venus, goddess of love, relies on Cupid's arrows to create new matches so that love does not disappear from the world, and so Cupid's stubborn refusal to fulfil his function risks both human procreation and, in consequence, the very tradition of glorifying Venus in gratitude for it. After months of stalemate, with nobody falling in love and no new life on earth, Venus realises she is being forgotten and the world is growing old, with the natural order broken down. It is Psykhe who is tasked with setting things right, and she undergoes a series of trials in the attempt. Sent into the underworld, Psykhe evades Cerberus, defeats a giant serpent, bests a host of other mythical beasts, and clears every obstacle placed before her, thereby proving her worth before the gods. She is finally reconciled with Venus, permitted to marry Cupid, and a drink of ambrosia secures mortal-born Psykhe's ascent to divinity. Together, Psykhe and Cupid then have a daughter – Hedone, the goddess of pleasure.

This story from antiquity, packed with supernatural themes, has provided the language now used to articulate our understanding of the mind. Every time we speak of psychology, psychiatry, psychosis, psychotherapy and the rest we invoke Psykhe's name. Her story is one that starts with love, and ranges through perilous enterprise, jealousy, despair, betrayal and forgiveness, before ending in growth to a higher state and, literally, the birth of blissful contentment. Psykhe's legend may not be the most famous amongst the ancient myths, but it is perhaps the most hopeful allegory for the arc of human progress.

I

A MODERN EPIDEMIC? – A PREMISE

The Book of Revelation describes four horsemen of the apocalypse, and they are all pretty scary. Conquest, War, Famine and Disease; a reminder of biblical proportions that we should have closed the stable door *before* the horses bolted. Perhaps the most menacing of all is the pale horse of Disease, the only one whose rider is named: '*It was death and Hell followed with him.*'[1] The pale horse has long stalked mankind. Before the nature of disease was understood, and when the means of curing or containing it remained unknown, epidemic outbreaks cut back the expansion of humanity with Malthusian regularity. As our forefathers first took to the seas, to travel and to trade, our first steps towards a connected world of immense social and economic possibilities were taken, but these networks also unleashed a darker possibility, that of pandemic – the rapid outbreak of disease across international borders.

Smallpox, cholera, influenza and the bubonic plague would become some of history's most prolific and brutal killers.

In the second century AD, soldiers returning from Mesopotamia introduced the 'Antonine Plague', thought to be smallpox, into the Roman Empire, where it is reckoned to have killed some five million[2] in the provinces of Greece, Asia Minor and Rome itself, wiping out whole communities. In the centuries that followed, outbreaks of bubonic plague communicated through trade routes across Asia, Europe and Africa, carrying away more than fifty million souls,[3] before cholera pandemics accounted for millions more in the eighteenth and nineteenth centuries, and the Spanish flu pandemic of 1918 claimed another fifty million.[4] These numbers are so great as to stagger comprehension. But whilst humanity's head was bloodied, it remained unbowed,[5] and scientific progress continued throughout. As the twentieth century progressed, a battery of advancements in pathology, immunology, sanitation and preventative medicine buttressed mankind against the charges of the pale horse. By 1980 the World Health Organisation was able to declare smallpox eradicated, and though a handful of cholera and bubonic plague fatalities are recorded each year even now, antibiotics and preventative controls had seemingly confined mass outbreaks to the history books. But the possibility of new, resistant pathogens exploding into being lurked ever in the background, and in 2020 the Covid-19 outbreak shattered our veneer of security. As it spread rapidly around the globe, uncertainty returned to life in a way that many of our ancestors knew, but most alive today could never previously have imagined. Humanity was once more forced to navigate extraordinary times, and Covid-19 was met with vigorous containment efforts. Extreme measures became normalised in very short order: the lockdown of many countries, the closure of workplaces and schools, and no expense spared as governments rushed to confront the threat; investing massive sums not just in health services, but in the de facto nationalisation of whole industries; underwriting private payrolls, and offering grants, loans and bailouts to make possible an unprecedented 'lockdown' to limit movement and limit transmission. These measures bought valuable time for health systems to marshal their resources, backed by governments that recognised the seriousness of the situation and responded proportionately. Yet Covid-19 is not the only illness to have presented such a clear and present threat to the health and lives of millions the world over in our times. There is another sphere of ill health with a reach and impact on a similarly massive scale; another sphere that the sophisticated arsenal of modern medicine has still barely begun to grasp, where our knowledge remains embryonic and our defences inadequate, and where our tolerance for accepting it seems curiously apathetic by comparison. It is mental ill health.

For more than a decade I was a Director of the UK's largest non-NHS provider of psychological therapies, and for six of those years held responsibility for the care of almost a hundred thousand patients each year – people referred to us by the National Health Service for help with depression, anxiety and other common mental health issues. Early in my tenure I was asked by a relative of the 'baby boomer' generation just what it was that we actually did.

'Mental health,' I answered.

'Mental health?' she replied, in a tone that made it clear that this was another question.

'We provide therapy for people struggling with their mental health.'

She looked at me like someone who had never heard the term, which I knew couldn't be true having just used it twice myself. She shook her head.

'There wasn't all that in my day.'

I remember wondering whether that could really be true. Were baby boomers comparatively untouched by mental health problems? Or were they present, but hidden and simply not discussed? Then, in 2017, on the occasion of the twenty-fifth celebration of World Mental Health Day, I wrote an article for the *Independent* newspaper that seemed to tap into a rich vein of recognition with readers. It turned on a few simple questions: '*Is mental ill health really a modern epidemic?*' '*If so then what is causing it?*' and '*Is modern life simply incompatible with good mental health for some people?*'

These are, of course, big questions. They require considerable unpacking, deserving much more than I was able to achieve in a short op-ed piece. Nevertheless, the central proposition – that we are experiencing a peculiarly modern crisis and that the structures of our globalised, digital world may be fuelling it – struck a chord with many. It was obvious that the question of whether there is an inherent mismatch between modern lifestyles and peace of mind was worthy of deeper exploration. Like a lawyer preparing arguments for the courtroom, we can readily erect a straw-man hypothesis. It runs like this: if human history is considered as twenty-four hours, the great majority of this time has been spent as pre-agricultural hunter-gatherers, and Christ only appeared around a quarter to midnight. Later still, finally escaping the age-old struggle for day-to-day survival, mankind had grown sufficiently in status and security to contemplate less visceral concerns. In the minutes before midnight humanity has raised its collective head, but doing so now surveys a bewildering vista of market forces charging to full expression: social media exploding into being, work-life balances increasingly unbalanced, and all in a world where the certainties and comforts once conferred by religion are ebbing away from ever more secular societies. This unprecedented combination of forces has crowded upon us with dizzying speed, crashing into human frailty and generating a reactionary tsunami of mental ill health. Today, one in four people will suffer a mental health issue in the course of each year.[6] Most will not seek help because of the stigma still attached to mental ill health, and after years in decline suicide rates among young people are now rising again.[7] This amounts to a desperate deposition of human suffering and of death. The old world catastrophes that harvested our ancestors have been replaced with something more insidious but just as fatal. It is not the inescapable death of plague, or the clamorous death of the battlefield; it is death by a thousand subtle cuts. Modern man barely registered being hanged, didn't notice getting drawn and can't recall being quartered, but he is dying all the same, and with silence on his lips.

After the World Mental Health Day article was published, I was taken aback by the response it generated – by the huge numbers of readers identifying with the suggestion that our modern, Western world is evolving more quickly than our human physiology and psychology can adapt to survive in it healthily. So, could the straw-man hypothesis be correct? Is today's high-octane lifestyle really less conducive to positive mental health than lifestyles used to be? On the surface this seems implausible. It may be a sweeping generalisation to say that the lot of the average person was worse in bygone centuries, but provided it is recognised to be such, a *generalisation* from which there are departures, it is a reasonable one to make. Whether a Bronze Age farmer with a life expectancy in the thirties, a production worker risking life and limb in an Industrial Revolution-era factory, a slave in one of the classical empires, or even one of their masters, the security and prosperity of the great majority would likely have been markedly *worse* in times past than the average person enjoys today. In modernity life expectancy, infant mortality and poverty are all trending favourably as never previously known, whereas life for all but the elite would have been grim enough to provoke misery as a rational response in most other periods of history. In this context we might intuitively expect to find that mental ill health issues are *less* prevalent now than in bygone days.

So the case for our straw man, if it is to be made, will not rest upon a narrative of how terrible life is today – comparatively speaking it *isn't*. But it will rely upon the premise of an innate conflict between the DNA of the human animal and the unique demands placed upon that animal in the modern world of sensory overload. The notion that there is something fundamental about human nature that renders us less well equipped to navigate the modern world in comparison with the world our predecessors knew – one that was poorer and more dangerous, but also more boundaried, and so perhaps more compatible with our processing capacity. Life in bygone times may have been short and brutal, but it may also have been better suited to our evolution. If so, there is a perverse sense in which a modern epidemic of mental health could even be regarded as a *good* thing – a negative side effect of positive progress. Are we witnessing the convulsions of maturity? Growing pains on the way to a better world? Perhaps current concern over society's mental health represents a high watermark of civilisation, a circumstance only available once basic social conditions have reached the critical threshold that permits the possibility. So in the mix of potent, pan-generational forces shaping modern life, just what is really going on? Are we in the grip of a modern epidemic? Have things always been this way? Or have the structures of twenty-first-century Western society created new conditions for mental health? Even new mental health conditions?

These questions will form our agenda, but answering them will be anything but straightforward. Historically, mental health has been a moveable feast. Whether or not a particular behaviour is considered normal or abnormal depends on the social context surrounding that behaviour – a fluid perception sighted from cultural conventions of the times. Some commentators have even argued that mental illness does not exist *at all*, but is merely a social construct used to articulate what happens when people simply being people behave in ways that jar with accepted norms to the point where it becomes convenient to attach a label to them, thereby categorising them under that label with others displaying similarly inconvenient behaviours. They assert that mental illness is over-medicalised, and that we are defining illness according to the degree of dissonance from average behaviour erroneously, when we are all just humans on a spectrum, exhibiting the natural rate of diversity present within the human condition. Whilst these arguments may have merits at the margins, the concept of psychiatric diagnoses as mere confected labels breaks down when we consider severe forms with a clear biological component, or the overwhelming evidence base now available that some psychological issues, like anxiety and depression, respond to treatment with good results.[8] In this light the claim that mental ill health is an immutable resting state warranting no intervention is like arguing that we should not bother exercising because it's human nature to sit on the couch, or not trouble to manage a diabetic's insulin levels because imbalances are normal within the human spectrum too. So, whilst we may acknowledge grey areas over where lines should be drawn, we must proceed from the generally accepted starting point that mental health is real and important, and actively looking after our mental health is important too.

This starting assumption does not allow us to escape the issue of definition, and amongst the arguments a defence counsel might array against the straw man, questions of definition and data must feature prominently. Mental ill health, just like physical ill health, takes many forms. Bipolar disorder is as different to obsessive-compulsive disorder as toothache is from typhoid. A broken nose is a broken nose – and often visibly so. But when cognitive processes drive a person to extraordinary behaviours, the act of correctly recognising them as symptoms of a psychological origin, grouping these symptoms together and then pinpointing a specific condition is not such a simple task. At coarse granularity we can separate off traumatic brain injury and biological neurodegenerative diseases like dementia outside the scope of these enquiries. Considering what *is* in scope, a distinction can also be drawn between severe and enduring mental health issues, like schizophrenia, and more moderate conditions such as anxiety or milder depression. It is these two that are by far the most common psychological issues, accounting for the great majority of today's one in four prevalence statistic. So, if there is a modern epidemic, then these conditions are crucial to it. But this complicates matters – moderate mental health issues are particularly difficult to track over time. In ages past, the withdrawn suffering associated with depression would have been more likely to pass unnoticed in comparison with conditions like schizophrenia, more likely to produce behaviours intruding into public attention. A certain level of collective altruism is necessary for mild to moderate mental health issues even to register with society. Beyond this difficulty there is also the need to distinguish between anxiety and depression as a natural and temporary response to the tribulations of life, as opposed to being a 'resting state', that impairs our ability to pursue that normal life. A little anxiety can be good for us; it is an evolutionary protection. It may be what drives us to think twice about big decisions, or to look before we leap, and everybody will feel a bit down sometimes. It is only when these feelings are prolonged beyond usefulness, becoming problematic, that they breach the diagnosis threshold. We should be careful not to attribute labels to passing reactions to events; we are all human and must all negotiate life's ups and downs. But precisely because we are all human, with our physical health, mental health, our work and social circumstances intertwined, the environments we inhabit and the events we experience *do influence* our individual mental health and the mental health in our societies. Crucially, this permits the possibility that changes in the character of our societies over time can either migrate towards, or away from, conditions optimised for nurturing mental well-being. Yet there is no historical master key to unlocking all secrets of the psyche. It was 1952 before a comprehensive classification of mental disorders, with common definitions that were broadly accepted across international boundaries, became available when the American Psychiatric Association published its *Diagnostic and Statistical Manual of Mental Disorders* (DSM), this first edition a somewhat bald enumeration of conditions that has been amended and added to ever since. Then in 1990 the *International Classification of Mental and Behavioural Disorders (ICD-10)* was endorsed at the forty-third World Health Assembly, before passing into common usage by World Health Organisation member states as of 1994. Whilst the construction of both indexes has attracted critique, these were important steps towards achieving common international definitions to help codify mental disorders, providing greater standardisation to better illuminate the depth of their prevalence, and thereby facilitating at least some possibility of scientific longitudinal analysis to help us understand whether our collective mental health really is getting worse.

Taking what evidence they could from the period for which good statistical data is available, the Institute for Health Metrics Evaluation's 2017 *'Global Burden of Disease'* report acknowledged a small ticking up of mental ill health since 1990.[9] Yet adjusted for population increase, the net rise is not of a scale that needs an epidemic to explain it, and could simply be a result of greater efforts to combat stigma in recent years – efforts that have helped people feel more comfortable reaching out to seek help, rather than struggling in secret and below the statistical radar. Moreover, because standardisation of mental health definitions has only existed in a meaningful way since the second half of the twentieth century, the time frame for which we have good statistical data is minuscule in the historical context. Statistics on mental health in recent decades tell us nothing conclusive about how the structures of modern society, evolved over centuries, facilitate mental health now in comparison with how the structures of centuries past did then. When the vast vista of recorded history is transposed onto that twenty-four-hour clock our empirical data begins mere seconds before midnight, and even now, with the act of diagnosis still largely dependent on people self-reporting their feelings, there remains considerable scope for subjectivity when medics attempt to work out which of many possible diagnoses might apply to each patient passing in front of them.

In summary, the available data is both severely limited and loaded with opportunity for statistical error. In this context attempts to make comparisons of mental health across gaping chasms of time, when the background noise of social and economic context has also markedly changed, must be heavily caveated. In the absence of reliable data any attempt to enumerate an exhaustive list of diagnoses and make comparisons with bygone ages, when some conditions we know today had not even achieved recognition, is to try and make bricks without straw – an ambition so fraught as to be futile as a scientific exercise. We do have richer information about past elites, benefitting from a wealth of contemporary sources covering all aspects of the lives of some privileged individuals. Speculating on the madness of King George, on whether Byron really was mad, or merely bad and dangerous to know, or revisiting the bloody records of notorious figures like Genghis Khan and Vlad Tepes through the medical lens, seeking to attach psychiatric diagnoses to notorious acts can be entertaining diversions.

Still, they are only diversions, because reading too much into such an exercise would be falling into another trap – that of judging old actions by new standards. Things were indeed different then, and a lifetime's conditioning so unique as to allow for no reference point in the modern world is bound to produce vivid results.

These caveats could serve as an argument for taking the modern age as ground zero for a study of mental health, but if our straw man was before the courts they would not stand up as an excuse for doing so. There is nothing new under the sun,[10] and it is by unfolding the past we can best understand how present attitudes to mental health were shaped. Whilst statistical data on inter-generational mental health prevalence may be unavailable, there is plenty of instructive material that is in scope. Cultures throughout the globe have recorded an abundance of anthropological detail about the people they relied on to farm their food, fight their battles and build their monuments. From the contours of history insights can be found on shifting attitudes to mental health, evolving interpretations of causation, and a few striking turning points that still cast a shadow over the shape of healthcare systems today. We also have a rich and at times horrifying record of methods attempted to 'cure' mental health issues, from the supernatural to the scientific. These are important insights because mental health is an issue we need to understand. In the unique circumstances of the modern world it feels we are wrestling at the sharp end of the eternal question – what does it truly mean to live well as a human? So, are we experiencing a modern mental health epidemic? The medical definition of the term is '*a widespread occurrence of a disease in a community at a particular time*', and whether or not things were better or worse way back when, in the here and now one in four certainly seems to qualify. The pale horse gallops on exalted.

2

THE EMANCIPATION OF REASON – MENTAL HEALTH IN THE ANCIENT WORLD

'*Those whom the gods destroy, they first make mad.*'[1] For the great majority of time that human beings have walked the earth, supernatural explanations dominated understanding of mental ill health, with blame for its symptoms attributed to spirits or demons. It was in classical times that naturalistic conceptions of causality first emerged to gain their bridgehead. The long, circuitous progression of human understanding through scientific, pseudoscientific, biological, psychological, and biopsychosocial theories of mental health was begun.

Supernatural Explanations for Mental Ill Health

Neolithic skeletons have been unearthed bearing evidence of trepanation – the practice of boring holes into the skull. The precise, regular nature of these holes suggests association

Psykhe

with attempted medicine, rather than battle or accidental injury, and the healing evident in specimens as much as 8,000 years old indicates that at least some patients survived their procedures. Weight of academic opinion is that these subjects were likely thought to be possessed by spirits, and the holes deemed the most pragmatic means of release. Trepanned skeletons have been discovered throughout Europe and the Americas, with concentrations in sites as diversely spread as France and Peru. We cannot know for sure what caused these trepanation subjects to be selected for their procedures, but it is a reasonable inference that some aberrance of behaviour marked them out, earning a place under the surgeon's knife – or flint as it probably would have been. Behaviour so jarring that their baffled contemporaries resorted to similarly extraordinary, supernatural explanations to make sense of it, leading to the same attempted remedies in consequence, but behaviour sufficiently common to the human condition that it affected a proportion of all cultures the world over. It may be that through these skulls we are seeing in the archaeological record some of the earliest attempts to manage mental ill health, albeit that it would not have been rationalised in those terms at the time. To modern minds a brutal procedure like trepanation sounds far removed from medicine, but perceptions of causation have always influenced choice of remedy. To someone convinced that a patient is shaking because of demonic possession, drilling the demon out may seem eminently rational.

Egypt was one old world civilisation that wholly subscribed to supernatural explanations for mental ill health. The Ancient Egyptian civilisation spanned many thousands of years and dozens of royal dynasties. Their culture invested special importance in beliefs in life after death, something that was sustained throughout. It is why the ruling pharaohs expended their subject's blood, sweat and lives so freely building pyramids, making the preparations needed for the afterlife. Upon death, Egyptians believed they would face the 'Judgement of Osiris', whereby their heart would be weighed in a scale balanced by a feather. This would ascertain the virtue in their souls, and so their worthiness to proceed to the afterlife. The Egyptian god of magic was also their god of medicine and the two concepts were intertwined close to unification in the minds of Ancient Egyptians, so that ill health, both physical and mental, was attributed to the gods. As a result, priests had an important role in healing and remedies typically involved incantations that were a hybrid of religious and medical in nature. Extraordinary insights into Egyptian attitudes have been preserved in a small number of medical papyri surviving from ancient times. Most valuable for an exploration of mental health are the *Ebers Papyrus*, the *Edwin Smith Papyrus*, the *London and Berlin Papyri*, the *Chester Beatty Medical Papyrus* and the *Carlsberg Papyrus*, probably the best papyrus in the world.

The *Ebers Papyrus* is divided into sections, ordering its contents according to recognisable fields of medicine. Grouped in this way is information on the alimentary system, the nervous system, the heart and circulatory system, diseases of the eyes, ears, nose and throat, and considerable material dedicated to surgery and even cosmetics – treatments to improve the appearance of skin and hair. It has no section dedicated to mental health, and it would be easy to infer that Ancient Egyptians were more concerned with wrinkles than well-being, but the perils of definition, always limiting when trying to grasp attitudes to mental health, are particularly acute when dealing with hieroglyphs. In Egypt the heart was considered the seat of the soul, and so heart and soul were translated as one, with consciousness, the mind and spirit all closely equated concepts. Egyptian comprehensions of the spark of life conflated with its beating heart.

The papyrus that would become named for him entered the possession of Egyptologist Edwin Smith in 1862, when he purchased it from an antiquities dealer in Luxor. It was 1930 before academics at the University of Chicago produced for the world a comprehensive translation of its contents. When they did so, established wisdom was not so much turned on its head, as exploded to shards. The papyrus devotes its main attention to war wounds, including head injuries and damage to the brain. Although rudimentary in places, it exhibits remarkable understanding of human physiology and the human body as a system – listing symptoms of injuries that would be felt far from the locus of damage. The papyrus is thought to be the product of multiple ancient hands, each adding notes on earlier contents successively over centuries, but the bulk is believed to have been written by the originator author at the time of the Old Kingdom, around 2,500 BCE – dating that came to light in 1930, when the earliest known medical writings on the brain were hitherto thought to have been those of Alcmaeon of Croton, made some two millennia later. Because the Edwin Smith papyrus demonstrates such detailed knowledge of injuries that might typically be incurred in battle, it has been suggested that the original author may have been a surgeon attached to the Egyptian army, accompanying them on campaign. Although no identification can be made with certainty, some academics have suggested Imhotep as a candidate,[2] legendary vizier to the twenty-seventh-century BCE Pharaoh Djoser, later deified as a god of medicine in both Egypt and Ancient Greece. Whilst the *Edwin Smith Papyrus* is by nature a treatise on physiological medicine, grounded in the biological world, it does not extend into anything recognisably psychological – having been written in a time when the seat of the sentient soul was still thought to have been the heart. At this time the brain, not needed for Osiris to reach judgement, was one of the organs routinely scooped out and discarded during mummification. Egyptians regarded brain matter as merely a redundant cranial stuffing, something considered only arguably true today, even in the case of politicians.

Nevertheless, the medical papyri provide insights about Egyptian treatments for maladies of all types, including some that sound psychological in nature, despite them not being understood in those terms at the time. The *Chester Beatty Papyrus* in particular is a glorious aggregation of prescriptions, bristling with remedies attempted by the ancient Egyptians. Because of the base association Egyptians made between religion and disease, magical incantations feature prominently, but dancing, painting, music and other social activities are also suggested for a range of disturbances that could have had a mental component, activities that a psychologist or mindfulness practitioner might recommend today – encouraging 'creative therapies' and opportunities for people in distress to draw peer support by socialising with others experiencing similar difficulties. In combination, the Egyptian texts throw up a curious mix of ideas that sound remarkably modern alongside some that seemingly confound. Motivated by their mistaken belief in divine causality, some Egyptian remedies were even designed to deliberately *worsen* the condition of the patient's body, in pursuit of an imagined greater good. Smearing excrement on patients, for example, is recommended in dozens of prescriptions in the *Ebers papyrus*, a treatment conceived of the same logic that led to trepanation – belief that the sufferer had been possessed. It was hoped that a debased human vessel, and the sickly, enfeebled corpus that might have resulted, would make a less attractive host for evil spirits to occupy, and that they would be driven out. The Egyptians may also have originated the belief that the uterus was prone to displace and wander around the body, causing hysteria in women, a conviction that lodged and transferred to Ancient Greek culture.

Early Natural Medicine in the Graeco-Roman World

In Ancient Greece too it was widely believed that ill health in general and mental disorders especially were bestowed by the gods. But this received wisdom was not a consensus, and from the polis cradle of democracy a small group of physicians and philosophers blazed the trail of enquiring science that would undergo centuries of buffeting, but ultimately vindicate their efforts. Alcmaeon of Croton performed some of the earliest recorded dissections and is often credited as first to identify the brain, rather than the heart, as the site of the mind, describing its critical role in the higher functions:

> All the senses are connected in some way with the brain. As a result, they are incapacitated when it is disturbed or changes its place, for it then stops the channels, through which the senses operate.[3]

Pinpointing the brain as the source of mental functioning is a breakthrough that seems so basic today that it might easily be underappreciated, but imagine being born into a world where it is not one of the givens taught in childhood, with no textbooks to help, and no brain imaging or other apparatus to reveal how the brain activates with stimuli. Is it just the fact that our eyes, granting our outlook onto the world, are located in our heads that suggests to us that the seat of reason lies directly behind? How would we know for sure? Not everyone did, but Alcmaeon advanced humanity that far at least in the fifth century BCE. Then the treatise *On the Sacred Disease*, written around 400 BCE and credited to the Hippocratic corpus, did much to disrupt the prevailing supernatural framework of health, arguing that people stricken with disease were not victims of divine machinations at all, but of natural, physiological causes:

> Men ought to know that from nothing else but the brain come joys, delights, laughter and sports, and sorrows, griefs, despondency, and lamentations ... And by the same organ we become mad and delirious, and fears and terrors assail us ... all these things we endure from the brain, when it is not healthy.[4]

The 'Sacred Disease' confounded ancient minds. It was said to generate symptoms of hysterical madness, shaking and frothing at the mouth, and it is thought today that the text refers to epilepsy. At the time its symptoms had reinforced supernatural beliefs held by many Ancient Greeks – with effects so terrible yet devoid of any observable, exterior trauma or injury to explain them, how could they not? Contemporary medical knowledge could offer no better explanation, and so it must have been easy to believe that these patients were receiving punishment from the gods. In the face of these strident opinions the Hippocratic text argued that the true cause of the Sacred Disease was really a build-up of phlegm in the brain, a claim rooted in Hippocrates' new framework of belief that *all* illness resulted from some imbalance in one or more of four bodily fluids – or humours. Humoral theory identified these as blood, phlegm, black bile and yellow bile. Excess black bile was thought to be responsible for depression and low mood – the word 'melancholy' derives from the Greek *'melaina kholé'*, literally 'black bile'. Surplus phlegm was associated with apathetic behaviour, as in 'phlegmatic', and was sometimes called the quiet mania. Surplus yellow bile was responsible for full-blown raging mania, extreme anger and agitation. Blood was believed to be produced by the liver and when in proper balance, uncontaminated by an excess of other humours, the result would be a content and sanguine nature accompanied by a positive, social and active lifestyle. Because humoral theory was predicated on the premise that imbalance of these fluids caused illness, the proper function of the physician shifted in response. Theirs became a task of restoring lost balance, with treatments like purging, starving and bloodletting following in corollary, interventions that remained common in mental health institutions millennia later.

Hippocratic teachings were widely adopted by Ancient Greek and Roman physicians, found still greater amplification in the writings of Galen, and became accepted wisdom amongst ancient world physicians. In this way and broadly speaking, physicians in classical times came to think of mental health disorders being divided into two types, melancholia and mania, occupying opposite poles on a spectrum that ranged between the excessively listless and excessively manic. Aretaeus of Cappadocia (AD *c.* 150–200), extending this thinking, has been credited with making the first description of what would eventually be called bipolar disorder, recording observations of patients who would endure long spells of melancholia interrupted by violent outbursts of mania, lurching rapidly between the two conditions at the spectrum's opposite poles. Whilst the concept of humorous imbalance as the cause of all ills may not have been correct, Hippocrates' ideas are not so far removed from modern-day notions of hormone dysregulation contributing to mental distress. There was, at least, no room for the gods in Hippocrates' medical philosophy. Though his humoral herring may have been as red as it was bilious, herrings of whatever colour reside indisputably in the natural world. The simple fact that Hippocrates' theory was wholly natural was, of itself, progress, and the reverence in which he is held today is rooted in Hippocrates' determination to reclaim medicine from the heavens, offering a comprehensive physiological architecture for understanding health that encompassed mental illness as well as physical. And, as the latter centuries BCE ticked down, an iteratively clearer conceptualisation of mental health as a distinct specialism in its own right, more than a mere aside to representations of health as a whole, unfolds in the ancient medical texts.

Alongside religion and nascent natural medicine, philosophy too was competing for classical hearts and minds as a framework through which people could understand the world, themselves and their well-being. A few decades after Hippocrates' death in 370 BCE, a new philosophical creed began to gather the popularity that would see it flourish throughout the Graeco-Roman world for some six centuries. The 'Stoics' are a group whose name remains synonymous with virtue, wisdom and composed endurance of hardship. Stoics held that virtue is the highest good, and can be attained by making peace with human nature, to achieve self-mastery in harmony with the rest of the natural world. Finding this 'ataraxia' would fortify the Stoic against life's inevitable ups and downs, which may test the emotions, but were immaterial to the Stoic, and to be met with dispassion. For them the concept of mental wellness was achieving contentment in the moment, not abstracted by anxiety about the future or the pursuit of base desires for pleasure or wealth. Some Stoics took this view to its extreme, regarding *any* emotion as a sign of mental disturbance, believing that dispassionate fortitude was essential to comprehending the universal reason, or 'logos'. Aristotle, whose ethical philosophy agreed closely with the Stoics, wrote *'Knowing yourself is the beginning of all wisdom.'*[5]

In the second century AD, when Stoicism was established as the dominant philosophy throughout Greece, physician Soranus of Ephesus wrote *'On Acute and Chronic Diseases'*. Although all originals were lost, Roman physician Caelius Aurelianus preserved a Latin translation. The work propelled classical thinking on mental health another leap forwards by finessing the coarse duopoly of mania and melancholy into a more detailed categorisation of mental disorders, fleshing out the distinctive characteristics that would help distinguish each one. Soranus nominated a third top-level categorisation of mental illness, adding phrenetis to mania and melancholia. Phrenetis was characterised by fever, fluctuating pulse and spasmic jerking. Soranus' conception of melancholia subdivided this hitherto baggy, umbrella diagnosis into its more moderate forms – a despondent but passing melancholy, as we might now associate with depression, and more severe manifestations, rising to prolonged paranoia and acute catatonic stupor. Mania, to Soranus, referred to delusion and extreme behaviour of a type that might today be associated with schizophrenia. His terminology did not correspond precisely with the many highly specified, modern diagnoses, but the rough shape of today's categorisation of mental illnesses can be perceived emerging from the fog. Soranus also offered up some remarkably sophisticated suggestions on treatment. He was an advocate of the simple power of speaking with people as a means of soothing their distress – an early trailblazer of the talking therapies. Familiar ideas about treatment are found too in the works of Asclepiades of Bithynia, now in modern-day Turkey, but part of the Roman Empire in the second century BCE. Asclepiades recommended exercise, fresh air, hydrotherapy and even music as treatments for mental disturbance and exhorted the importance of a good diet to preventing mental illness and maintaining a positive mindset. These progressive views earned many admirers, but in Rome as in Egypt, early attempts to wrestle with mental health also produced misfires. The theory that mental ill health is caused by low morals dates to Cicero, a contemporary of Asclepiades. According to Cicero, a colossus of the age whose standing owes nothing to his ruminations on mental health, serious mental illnesses were inflicted by the 'Furies' – goddesses of Hades – on their victims.

> The punishments they undergo are not so much those inflicted by courts of justice, as what they suffer from conscience. The furies pursue and torment them, not with their burning torches, as the poets feign, but by remorse, and the tortures arising from guilt... It is a man's own dishonesty, his crimes, his wickedness, and boldness, that takes away from him soundness of mind; these are the furies, these the flames and firebrands, of the wicked.[6]

By compromising themselves through immoral deeds Cicero believed people condemned themselves to madness. He coined the term 'Furens' to describe the disturbances inflicted as punishment – the torment of acting in conflict with conscience. 'Insania' was Cicero's description for the milder mental malaises which, he believed, had no divine originator, but were symptoms of excess emotion and lack of wisdom. Neither idea added many cubits to his reputation.

Mental Illness in Classical Literature

As the great classical works track down antiquities passing centuries, attitudes to mental health can be seen evolving on their pages, as shifting conceptions carry through into classical literature. The cast of human heroes that decorate Homer's *Iliad* and *Odyssey*, written in the eighth century BCE, are characters of action, but limited agency. Mostly they are puppets in the hands of the gods, their fates decided on the whims of superior, supernatural forces, as they are swept along on waves of circumstance never comfortably within their control. At the *Iliad*'s climax Ajax is driven to madness by the goddess Athena, and in his delusions slaughters a flock of sheep, believing them, under Athena's influence, to be enemy soldiers. Once Ajax regains his senses his shame at actions committed whilst deprived of them leads him to commit suicide. He considers himself dishonoured, and the dishonour is unbearable. Ajax is mortal man capable of powerful emotions, but remains a plaything of the gods, ravaged to destruction by superior forces.

By the fifth and fourth century BCE Sophocles and Euripides were animating their characters with richer humanity than the puppets filling the pages of the *Iliad* and *Odyssey* – although they typically fared little better. Sophocles' *Oedipus Rex* sees the titular King of Thebes become the subject of a prophecy that he will murder his father, King Laius, and sleep with his mother. Learning of this premonition, Laius orders the infant Oedipus executed, but Oedipus survives the attempt, is taken in by adoptive parents and grows to adulthood ignorant of both the prophecy and his true parentage. When he does learn of it, Oedipus takes every precaution to escape his fate, leaving home to put distance between himself and his adopted parents. But these efforts only set the stage for the prophecy's fulfilment, when Oedipus unknowingly encounters his birth father Laius on his travels and kills him in a quarrel. When he learns the truth, Oedipus is overwhelmed, gouging out his own eyes in his torment. Sophocles' depiction of Oedipus is one of flawed humanity wrestling with destiny, and its power lies in the psychological anguish he endures. Ultimately Oedipus is unable to escape his divined fate, but there is plenty of human emotional turmoil as he agonises over the attempt. The rounded complexity of Oedipus' persona finds expression inside the Graeco-Roman paradigm of the gods, with no inherent incompatibility between the two. Naturalistic depictions of mental distress, often in response to extreme events, and supernatural depictions – mental health inflicted directly by displeased deities – were now co-existing in a delicately balanced dance, often in the very same stories.

This interplay of supreme manoeuvrings and human nature is showcased again in the story of Psykhe herself, another goddess of Greek mythology. Her name means *'breath of life'*, but in Psykhe the vital spark received more than human personification; it was given divine form as the goddess of the soul. Psykhe's story describes her birth as a mortal woman and long struggle to be united with her love – Cupid, son of the goddess Venus. Envious of Psykhe's beauty and abetted by Psykhe's equally jealous sisters, Venus throws herself into a campaign to keep the lovers apart, and Psykhe is forced to undergo a series of trials that rival the labours of Hercules. Sent into the underworld by Venus, she confronts Cerberus, a giant serpent and even some killer sheep – very different to the benign creatures attacked by Ajax. Psykhe is resolute in the face of all. After Venus sets her the seemingly impossible task of separating a large basket of mixed grains an ant takes pity on Psykhe and, with an army of friends, completes the trial for her in an inspired touch of pre-Disney Disney. After navigating every obstacle Venus can muster, Cupid and Psykhe are eventually summoned to Mount Olympus to meet with Zeus, who grants the lovers permission to marry. A drink of ambrosia secures Psykhe's ascent to divinity and Venus forgives her new daughter-in-law. Together Psykhe and Cupid have a daughter – Hedone, the goddess of pleasure whose name is now the basis of 'hedonism'. Psykhe has had an enduring legacy; the etymology of our modern English 'Psychology' and its many familial derivations are a portmanteau of Psykhe's name and the Greek word '*logos*' ('logia' in Latin), meaning speech, reason or logic. Thus, a myth from ancient times, packed with the customary gods, goddesses and the supernatural themes, also tackles issues of mortal emotion and humanity's complex internal responses to external trials, providing the language that today describes the scientific understanding of the mind.

So what does this classical curate's egg of mythology and medicine tell us about mental health in antiquity? The impression is one of gathering progressive forces amidst a scattergun suite of ideas, simmering together in civilisations still largely hamstrung by a common, first principles impediment – widespread belief in supernatural causation. Nevertheless, there is clear evidence from ancient times that at least some people understood the brain as the site of cognitive processing, with a developing and increasingly nuanced concept of mental illnesses beyond obvious and acute 'madness', recognising conditions like transient melancholia, that we might equate with mild to moderate depressive issues today. So we know too that the existence of lower-level issues, those that today constitute the great majority of the suggested modern epidemic, was at least acknowledged, even in classical times. Evident too is appreciation of the need to care for our emotional well-being, and some understanding of intrinsic links between environmental and social factors, our lifestyles, our diets and our state of mind. Portentous ideas about treatment were also blossoming in some quarters of the ancient world, early experiments with interventions that might just about qualify as talking therapy, group therapy, peer support or mindfulness in modern parlance; treatments that were infinitely more humane than the previously conventional alternatives – locking people away or simply abandoning them to destitution. The potential of music to stir emotions and lift the soul was also well understood, and may be why the Egyptian texts, along with equivalents from Babylonia and Assyria, often recommended that their healing incantations should be sung or chanted in the presence of patients.

In this hotbed of ancient ideas the new, naturalistic theories of mental ill health were quickly finding their place alongside the supernatural ones that had prevailed from time immemorial. Though they had not yet achieved the expulsion of supernatural thinking from medicine, the popularity of natural beliefs was growing on a trajectory that seemed to promise an eventual triumph of reason over superstition. But for that, there would be a long wait. Concepts of mental ill health as divine punishment or demonic possession would soon be resurgent, reasserting primacy as the Roman Empire fell into decline. As it did so the flickers of ancient progress would be snuffed out, and human understanding stalled for centuries, when the glory and the grandeur of the classical world gave way, and Europe plunged into the Dark Ages.

3

BAYING AT THE MOON – RELIGION AND MENTAL HEALTH

'In the beginning God created the heavens and the earth'[1] – Genesis in a particularly parsimonious nutshell. But where to begin when it comes to the great questions of theology and their impact on our mental health? One option is to lump religion together with politics and money and not discuss it at all, but these are the major forces that have shaped the world as we know it, so we must venture into all three subjects in the coming chapters.

The Ascent of Christianity

We have seen how supernatural explanations for mental ill health dominated the ancient world whilst falling short of exclusivity; many Graeco-Roman philosophers and physicians were clear that mental illnesses had exclusively natural origins, and some worked actively to propagate this secular understanding. Yet these remained times when atheism was near non-existent, when almost every citizen would have subscribed to belief in whatever gods were sanctioned by the ruling powers in their part of the world. In this context it was religious paradigms that formed the fallback architecture helping people make sense of their lives, providing the moral compass and explanatory narrative that anchored them, and determining their relationship with the world they inhabited.

It was normal for old world cultures to have room for many gods, as was famously the case in both Greece and in Rome. Zeus, or Jupiter, may have been seated proudly at the head of the table, but the company was fulsome, with a multitude of minor gods, titans and muses responsible for everything from war to wealth and music to wine. No single deity held absolute claim over human reverence to the exclusion of all others. Even when Socrates found himself sentenced to death on trumped-up charges of 'impiety', or failing to respect the state gods, it was really political discomforts he had provoked, not reasons of religion, that saw him condemned. It was perhaps this relative religious tolerance that left the supernatural door sufficiently ajar to admit the chinks of scientific light that Hippocrates, Galen and others had begun to shine onto medicine. But the divine pecking order was about to be overhauled, and the old world gods replaced in a changing of the guard. Writing in the 1770s, the English Member of Parliament and historian Edward Gibbon described how the slow rise of a new religion coincided with the Roman Empire's decline:

While that great body was invaded by open violence, or undermined by slow decay, a pure and humble religion gently insinuated itself into the minds of men, grew up in silence and obscurity, derived new vigour from opposition, and finally erected the triumphant banner of the Cross on the ruins of the Capitol.[2]

In this way Christianity established a pre-eminent position throughout Europe. After years of intermittent state persecution of Christians, Emperor Constantine sanctioned the Edict of Milan in AD 313, granting them legal freedoms throughout a changing Roman Empire already in decline. The edict was a loosening of the noose that meant Christians no longer had to worship underground, and the Coliseum's lions were forced to broaden their palates. Through the following centuries invigorated Christianity assumed profound influence over the lives of millions of Europeans. And its teachings did not permit room for other gods, or indeed the worship of any 'false idols'. There was no space either for harmonious coexistence with philosophies of reason, or balance with the natural world, as had been the case with the religions of antiquity. Instead, fervour and unquestioning zeal characterised these early Christians – it was faith that mattered, not reason. In time, Christendom would spread to the Americas, Australia, Africa and other territorial possessions as the frontiers of European colonialism extended throughout the world, its missionaries carrying forth the gospels of hellfire and damnation, sacrifice and salvation. As Christianity flourished the Bible and the teachings of Christ replaced the myths of old world gods as the new bedrock of belief, establishing the parameters governing how people thought about their lives, and their health, for more than a thousand years. This was the Dark Age period of stagnation and the Established Church was at least partly responsible for the stultification of scientific and medical advancement that characterised it, often making deliberate interventions to this purpose. Tenth-century Pope Boniface the Seventh issued an edict banning autopsies – a rule strictly enforced – and the religious dictate *'the church abhors the shedding of blood'* was interpreted broadly by many as prohibiting not just violence, but any invasive medicine that might otherwise have advanced scientific knowledge. These attitudes interrupted medical progress in general, and mental health was no less a victim. Nevertheless, there is compelling evidence that the impact of Christendom on mental health in Western culture, through its long centuries of domination, has been complex, rather than uniformly bad.

Western Secularism

With due respect to the Jedi, Christianity is today generally considered one amongst the small group of great world religions – Islam, Hinduism, Buddhism, Sikhism and Judaism – the major faiths that, between them, count the overwhelming majority of the world's population as adherents. Over the centuries, the fortunes of each have inevitably shifted, but with the possible exception of state atheism in China, it is in the Western world where proportions of the faithful have altered most markedly in recent times, firstly as Christianity weathered the buffetings of science and Darwinism, and then in the wake of a frontal assault from the new god of capitalism – money. In many

Western European democracies, and in places like the United States and Australia where fundamentally similar values are shared, the trend of the last century has been towards increasingly secular societies.[3] A hard core of evangelicals remains amongst our religious communities, but among many who self-identify as Christian, the resting pulse ardour of faith has declined. In the twenty-first century attending a Church of England school, for instance, may mean hymns in assembly and an annual nativity production; it does not necessarily mean the same vigorous, blood and thunder devotion that was central to the lives of ancestors who lived and breathed their faith,[4] many so piously that they would sooner burn at the stake than compromise or recant it, as was the fate of some amidst the Catholic–Protestant denominational clashes that scarred the reigns of 'Bloody Mary' and Elizabeth I. This softening of faith has been accompanied by – arguably part-caused by – huge changes that have altered the texture of our societies – industrialisation, the ascent of capitalism, immense leaps in technology and a digital revolution amongst them. In the twentieth and twenty-first centuries this has distinguished the Western world from other cultures; whilst this combination of dynamics is not exclusive to the west, it is there that it has found fullest expression at the head of the curve. In modernity, financial indicators have become a default method for evaluating status and success. Our salaries are a value placed on the worth of our labours; our income brackets the determinant of the houses we live in, the cars we drive and the holiday destinations from which we upload photos for others to see. Past generations also had to worry about money of course, but their higher rates of religious belief, with associated spiritual measures of human value, kept the economic ones from achieving such sweeping dominance. As all this has happened, as capitalism has evolved into its globalised, digital age and as Western society has become more secular, a financially oriented mainspring of ideas has mimicked the path trodden by Christianity to insinuate its way into received wisdom. But has this model robbed us of space to breathe? Caused us to forget the questions that transcend materiality and remind us of what it means to live well? *'What is my purpose in life?' 'What is the value of my own being?' 'What is my duty to others?'* Has the light in our souls diminished just a bit? If waning belief has denuded an anchoring source of strength, we may have isolated the first ingredient fuelling a modern proliferation of mental ill health.

After all, there is comfort in abdicating responsibility for setting the rules of the game to a higher power; in outsourcing our thinking about justice, morality and what is right and wrong. For those who subscribe to a religion and adhere to its commandments, decisions on personal action often hold less anxiety. With rules for accessing the kingdom of heaven, it is a higher law that is to be followed, not day-to-day impulses or desires. Should I steal my neighbour's Ox? Well, no, because thou shalt not steal, of course, or covet thy neighbour's ox for that matter. There might be weightier moral dilemmas awaiting us on life's procession, but the peace of mind benefits accruing from sincerely held beliefs in a moral codebook are obvious, particularly when those convictions are reinforced by a community of like-minded people, and pastoral care when needed. When that certainty is lost, what happens next? Having reclaimed ownership of life's narrative, how should it be written? Into the void each individual must apply themselves to tasks previously reserved for God, and find their own metaphysical philosophy, perhaps something conducive to a healthy life, but perhaps instead an obsessive pursuit of wealth, of 'likes', of the bottle, or the needle. And for those who don't want to invent their own replacement philosophy, Darwin has one oven-ready – life as competition: short, brutal and often senseless; nature red in tooth and claw. So having cast off religion, what measure of comfort has it really been to witness the truth unvarnished, with scales gone from secular eyes? What victory is it to replace ignorance, when ignorance was bliss? Perhaps Pyrrhic, perhaps little has been gained, but paradise lost. We are naked and only just realising it.

Without faith, gone too is that mental serenity that trust in a higher power can bring to believers, whether we think they are correct in their convictions or not. If an omniscient divinity trumps all, what reason can there be for anxiety? It's all God's plan. The Bible contains many injunctions to adopt these comforting convictions. In Philippians 4:6-7:

> Be anxious for nothing, but in everything by prayer and supplication with thanksgiving let your requests be made known to God. And the peace of God, which surpasses all comprehension, will guard your hearts and your minds in Jesus Christ.[5]

And in Isaiah 41:10:

> Do not fear for I am with you; Do not anxiously look about you, for I am your God I will strengthen you, Surely I will uphold you with my righteous hand.[6]

The comforts of religion are also self-evident when the faithful find themselves bereaved, or trembling on the edge of eternity themselves, and are able to draw strength from their sure and certain hope in the resurrection to eternal life. Without it, scope for anxiety and despair is all the greater. Committed atheists might consider a chain of reasoning that correlates increasing mental ill health with decreasing rates of belief in a delusion to be ironic. It may be, but the rush towards secularism may nevertheless have seen us throw a particularly cherubic-looking baby out with the bathwater.

Psychotherapy and religion have long had an uneasy relationship. Publicly funded mental health services in particular, keen to favour no faith above any other, have often preferred to separate religion from care altogether, treating it like a hot potato, neglecting opportunities to leverage the fortification believers can derive from faith to the benefit of their treatment. Religious doctrine has been accused of fomenting negative mental health. Freud called religion a 'collective neurosis'. An avowed Darwinist, God had no place in Freud's psychoanalytical philosophy. He considered doctrinal pressure to observe strict routines objectionable, finding similarities between obsessive, compulsive pathology and the ritualistic behaviour encouraged by some faiths. The concept of 'religious stress' describes the anxiety that can accompany the rigorous practices of some denominations, particularly those that worship a punishing, rather than a benign, God. Nevertheless, the message of most religions is one of hope and people of faith generally consider their beliefs a source of sustenance. Religion has provided huge numbers of people with strength and fortification in times of hardship – the comforting feeling of being connected to something bigger than themselves; and reduction in faith has, broadly speaking, corresponded with rising awareness of mental ill health in the modern age. A relationship beyond coincidence is plausible, and the recent trend for secularism might just have removed one of the factors formerly safeguarding us against the proliferation of a mental health crisis.

Witchcraft and Possession

Religious ideation has also provided some of the most florid causal theories and 'remedies' for mental ill health conceived throughout history. The Old Testament book of Daniel offers a direct example of madness inflicted as divine punishment, as Babylonian King Nebuchadnezzar is driven from his senses for taking excessive pride in his own majesty:

> At that moment the sentence against Nebuchadnezzar was fulfilled. He was driven away from mankind, and he began to eat vegetation just like bulls, and his body became wet with the dew of the heavens, until his hair grew long just like eagles' feathers.[7]

The eternal struggle raging between the Devil and the Holy Spirit for possession of the human soul is a primary tenet of Christian belief, and the New Testament too has several accounts of demonic possession. In Mark 5:1 Jesus encounters an unfortunate man occupied by an 'unclean spirit'. The man is described as living roughly, terrorising his neighbours and even self-harming until Jesus casts the spirit out:

> Then they came to the other side of the sea, to the country of the Gadarenes. And when He had come out of the boat, immediately there met him out of the tombs a man with an unclean spirit, who had his dwelling among the tombs; and no one could bind him, not even with chains … always, night and day, he was in the mountains and in the tombs, crying out and cutting himself with stones. When he saw Jesus from afar, he ran and worshipped Him. And he cried out with a loud voice and said, 'What have I to do with You, Jesus, Son of the Most High God? I implore You by God that You do not torment me.' For He said to him, 'Come out of the man, unclean spirit!'[8]

The capacity of evil spirits to invade the human corpus, bringing madness when they do, is cited again in Mark, 5:9-13. Another man describes multiple malevolent personalities occupying his body and tells Jesus, '*My name is legion, for we are many,*' before the many are promptly dispatched into a herd of swine and driven into the sea by an unimpressed Messiah. Many Christian denominations have adopted literal interpretations of these passages, believing that the service Jesus provided to the afflicted was not merely inspiration to change their ways, or some other metaphorical liberation, but the expulsion from their bodies of an actual foreign invader. The cliché Hollywood image of possession is one of a demented sufferer with arms reversed in their sockets, eyes bulging and breath steaming the air. But in the real world the behaviours exhibited in suspected possession cases were often of a type that might be associated with schizophrenia, epilepsy, or psychosis today. For most of history these conditions remained misunderstood, unknown to the canon of medical knowledge, and unmolested by its physician practitioners. Into this void supernatural explanations for the symptoms exhibited were proposed, accepted and acted upon with few misgivings.

Belief in witches and in witchcraft as an explanation for abnormal or eccentric behaviour was common throughout the Middle Ages. By the sixteenth century, it was so widespread that the English parliament was obliged to legislate for it. The Witchcraft Act of 1542 created an offence of witchcraft, punishable by death, and James VI of Scotland even wrote a book on the subject – *Daemonologie*, published in 1597. This was just six years before Queen Elizabeth died and James also became King James I of England, so his keen interest in witchcraft was a strong establishment endorsement for fervid clerical voices convinced that the devil was working amongst them. When James assumed the English throne his new subjects suddenly found it expedient to sympathise with these views and belief in witchcraft boomed. The strength of James' feelings about witches was rooted in experiences that already dated back some fifteen years by the time he was crowned in England. In 1589 he had travelled to Denmark ahead of his marriage to Princess Anne, sister of the Danish king. The outbound journey was uneventful, but afterwards James and Anne embarked on the return trip to Scotland under leaden skies. Their ship was beset by storms and James was forced to shelter in a Norwegian port to wait out the weather. A Danish official with the travelling party convinced James that this misfortune was the work of a network of witches in Scotland and Denmark and witch trials quickly followed in both countries. James located his trials in Berwick, where torture was routinely employed as a means of gaining confessions and, more perniciously, the names of co-conspirators from suspects. Under its threat both were readily forthcoming. Two supposed witches were quickly burned in Denmark and James' own investigations in Berwick grew to include more than a hundred suspected witches. One of them, Agnes Sampson, was brought before James in person to answer charges of conspiring to sink his ship by raising storms with black magic. Sampson initially refused to confess and was beaten, deprived of sleep and forced to wear a scold's bridle – an iron muzzle equipped with a spiked mouth plate to press the tongue. When Sampson eventually cracked her confession was complex and detailed, perhaps in hopes of securing a quick death in preference to further tortures. She admitted her participation in a witch coven that had connived with the devil to sink his ship and kill the King, describing her attempts to obtain an item of James' clothing for this purpose. She elaborated on the powdered animal bones used in her spells and curses, the cat she had drowned in the sea to raise the storm and occasions when the devil had visited her in the form of a dog in the course of the plotting. James had her garrotted and burned at the stake.

Shakespeare drew inspiration from Berwick, borrowing aspects for his tragedy *Macbeth*, also set in Scotland and first performed in 1606, two years after James' accession to the English throne. It is impossible to read *Macbeth* without being struck by the parallels between the practices unearthed during James' trials and Shakespeare's presentation of the three witches, or 'weird sisters', in the first scene of the first act. Shakespeare endows his witches with the power of loosing winds to raise storms; to them 'fair is foul and foul is fair' as they meet upon 'blasted heath' amidst thunder and lightning. The description Shakespeare places into Macbeth's mouth reads like a direct nod to Berwick:

> Though you untie the winds, and let them fight
> Against the churches; though the yesty waves
> Confound and swallow navigation up;
> Though bladed corn be lodged, and trees blown down;
> Though castles topple on their warders' heads[9]

The play's description of witches raising winds cannot have failed to ring unhappy bells for James, or most contemporaries witnessing a performance. Likewise, the image of castles toppling cannot have been a comfortable one for a king with good cause to be uneasy just months after the narrowly averted Gunpowder Plot. Back then, well before radio or television, Shakespeare's play, along with the endorsement of a King, would have constituted the best publicity imaginable for those arguing that witchcraft was a real possibility and a serious problem, propagating fear and loathing ever more widely.

Witch frenzy reached its fevered zenith in the early seventeenth century with the ugly career of Matthew Hopkins, remembered to history as England's Witchfinder General. Hopkins' fleeting infamy coincided with the English Civil War and he is thought to have been responsible for the execution of more than a hundred alleged witches, all terminated with extreme prejudice in a short period between 1643 and 1647. It is unclear whether Hopkins carried on his activities under the aegis of official parliamentarian sanction, but mandated or not the Witchfinder General pursued his mission with demonic energy, perhaps owing to the large sums he was able to command for his services – fees typically paid on a *per capita* basis of head of discovered witch. The generous financial rewards available may also explain why Hopkins was willing to sail perilously close to the limits of the law with the practices he employed when seeking confessions. If he spotted a belt, Hopkins aimed below it. It was he who devised the notorious water test, whereby suspects were tied and thrown into deep water, done on the theory that witches, having renounced their baptism, would be rejected by the water in return and by floating well enough to survive would reveal their guilt. Anyone accepted by the water, to the extent that they drowned, was declared innocent – although amnesty would likely have been little consolation as their lungs filled with water and life ebbed away. Armed with these tactics, Hopkins and his company travelled from town to town through the Puritan, Parliamentarian strongholds of southern England, seeking out witches, each one effectively waving a little cheque ready for him to bank on achieving their demise. Any eccentric behaviour he encountered must have been a great convenience for Hopkins as he grew wealthy under the specious cover of God's work – a devil quoting scripture for his own purposes. In 1647, a mere three years after accusing his first witch, with his methods under increasing scrutiny and perhaps sensing providence sneaking up behind him with the lead piping, Hopkins retired to a well-feathered nest in the country where he promptly contracted tuberculosis and died. He was not yet thirty and though Hopkins' end was less gruesome than that he inflicted on his victims, those hundred souls might yet have rested a little easier for his passing.

Reports of witches and witchcraft were common not only in Britain, but throughout Europe and the Americas too. One notorious case occurred in France when Bishop Charles Miron investigated the supposed possession of Martha Brossier, a young French woman, in 1600. Brossier was said to be suffering convulsions, speaking in tongues and using voices that were not her own. It was even claimed that she had been levitating. Miron was sceptical and devised a series of experiments to test these claims. Firstly he induced Brossier to drink holy water by passing it off as normal water. When this produced no effect, when one might have been expected in a genuine case, Miron presented Brossier with a purported holy relic, which was in fact a worthless prop, while reciting Virgil in hopes the verses might be mistaken for holy rites. Miron was staging a mock exorcism, and when it agitated an acute bout of Brossier's symptoms – minus the levitation presumably – he was satisfied that he had proved a deception. In many ways this makes Brossier's case even more puzzling. Here was someone who may have been suffering a psychological condition, approximating the symptoms of possession and being disbelieved by the supposedly sane on account of her condition not being supernatural enough. Quite the riddle. The obvious perils of being a suspected witch meant that most confessions had to be secured through torture. An unsolicited disclosure, or a pretence like Brossier's, seemed unfathomable, tantamount to a death wish – yet Brossier's is not a unique case.

Many theories have sought to explain the explosion of possession cases in the seventeenth and early eighteenth centuries. Many accused witches would simply have been unfortunate victims; in the wrong place at the wrong time, and on the wrong end of baseless accusations without merit, rhyme or reason. But many others would likely have been suffering some form of mental health issue by today's understanding. Another prosaic possibility is that simple material expedience may even have led some to *invite* accusations, where they might otherwise never have been made. People with wretched lives and little prospect of better might snap and act out in the only context they understood – through religion. This would have carried risks, but might also have elevated someone from the status of an anonymous, miserable peasant to that of someone *known*, someone to be feared and wondered at. Counterintuitive as it may be, in the context of an ultra-devout society, being considered a witch could have enhanced one's status, and certainly would have enhanced one's notoriety. No amount of perverse celebrity is any good if you're dead, of course, but not all convictions for witchcraft resulted in the death penalty.

Another theory is that cases of witchcraft were catching, going viral to the point where some people convinced themselves they really *were* witches. This was made possible by the strict religious conventions defining life at this time, which may have distorted psychological processes in insular and extreme communities. It was in the late sixteenth century that Puritan beliefs spread rapidly through England and America. Puritans thought that the Established Church had drifted from the literal word of the Bible, becoming fat and indulgent. They didn't just talk the talk, they walked the walk too, eliminating from their lives all luxuries and practices not expressly endorsed by the Bible, restoring God to centre stage. The word of God was both literal and final, and the social esteem Puritans accorded fellow members of society was determined by the perceived purity and depth of a person's faith. In this pressure-cooker environment, devotion approached competition. These conditions entrenched belief in the possibility of possession as a literal biblical truth, and in so doing, may have propagated psychotic episodes. In this suffocating atmosphere, what form could it take when someone found themselves pushed beyond endurance? All rebellion, by definition, is an act in opposition to the orthodoxy. If the orthodoxy is puritanical belief in God, the opposite is clear. For people like Martha Brossier, reared in ardent piety, there could be no more extreme rejection of her lot in life than to ally with the devil. As with Brossier's, most possession cases occurred in isolated areas with especially extreme devotion to biblical teachings, and detached from outside counterbalances. In modern psychological parlance, 'scrupulosity' is the term used to describe the compulsion or guilt that can lead us to obsess over observing correct behaviour – sometimes to the extent where we become *so afraid* of doing something wrong that we do something wrong, an unconscious mechanism for releasing the tension. In the modern world this could manifest as behaviour society might consider socially or politically incorrect, similar to a Tourette's sufferer involuntarily shouting obscenities. In the seventeenth century, when being politically correct was synonymous with being religiously correct, it might have manifested in blasphemy.

All the classic ingredients were present in America's most well-known series of witch trials, which would unfold to become one of the most woeful episodes in all American history. These were held in Massachusetts, in the little settlement of Salem, a township that would be propelled into infamy by the events that took place there between 1692 and 1693. At this time the England of William and Mary was at war with France over the North American colonies, and this 'Nine Years War' was partly fought in those colonies, causing much hardship to communities there, steeped in Puritan faith. Salem's descent to catastrophe began when the daughter and niece of Reverend Samuel Parris, the village minister, simultaneously began to experience fits of shaking, screaming, sobbing uncontrollably and throwing their bodies into seemingly impossible contortions in outbursts so violent that locals became convinced they must have had diabolical causes. Their doctor agreed, and the suggestion that their symptoms were the work of witches went from speculation to accepted fact with a speed and ease that could perhaps only have been possible in such an isolated, religiously fervent community. Under pressure from local magistrates, the girls pointed the finger at three vulnerable women: two destitute beggars and the Parris family's Caribbean slave. The three accused were quickly imprisoned, but paranoia that the devil was abroad in Salem was already rampant. The town became a snake pit of suspicion, and a slew of copycat allegations flooded the town in the following months, compelling Governor William Phipps to convene a special court dedicated to hearing the cases of Salem's alleged witches and pronouncing judgement upon them. Ultimately some two hundred were tried on accusations of witchcraft and twenty had been condemned to death by the time the court's proceedings concluded. Nineteen were hanged on the notorious 'Gallows Hill' and the twentieth, a man of more than eighty years, suffered a dreadful end pressed to death beneath heavy stones.

By the time the witch craze subsided, tens of thousands of innocent Europeans and Americans, mostly women, are thought to have lost their lives as a result of it.[10] By the mid-eighteenth century growing public distaste for court actions against alleged witches, increasingly recognised as being just vulnerable, unfortunate people, crystallised into law when Parliament in Britain repealed the Witchcraft Act in 1736. Although occasional instances of witch hunting and even witch killing persist in some corners of the globe, it has been centuries since any state has sanctioned an execution for witchcraft in the Western world. The modern Catholic Church still officially maintains both a literal belief in the possibility of possession and a staff of exorcists ready to carry on the implied workload, but a priest confronted today with a parishioner claiming literal possession is far more likely to nudge them in the direction of conventional medicine than invoke the exorcist's services. In a 2002 address Pope John Paul II spoke of spiritual combat in carefully subtle terms as 'a secret and interior art, an invisible struggle in which monks engage every day against the temptations, the evil suggestions that the demon tries to plant in their hearts'.[11] Opinion among many Christian, even Catholic clergy, is now that demonic possession has more currency as a metaphorical concept than a literal truth, albeit that this is a wisdom that sometimes remains unspoken and without final official sanction.

Faith Fostering Well-being?

Alternative religious narratives for making sense of the universe are, of course, available. The records of some are less blemished when it comes to producing the conditions in which good mental health is most able to thrive. Buddhism is one faith heavily associated with a positive mentality. Buddhists devote their lives to escaping the cycle of death and rebirth through attainment of Nirvana, reached through achieving enlightenment – a mental state of peaceful equilibrium. The meditative practice of *dhyana* involves narrowing the mind's attention to a single focal point, such as the rhythm of breath or a specific thought or mental image. Having enjoyed centuries of popularity with Buddhists, this technique has also recently become fashionable in Western societies under the alternative title of mindfulness. Hindus, too, believe in a cycle or birth, life, death and rebirth, and pursue a spiritual quest to transcend it. Hinduism defines four *Puruṣārthas* as the proper goals of life: *Dharma*, living according to moral values and duties; *Artha*, achieving prosperity through work; *Kama*, satisfying desires and passions; and *Moksha*, achieving release from the cycle of death and rebirth. Hindus worship, meditate, strive to optimise their karma and follow the yogas, pursuing lifestyles that they believe will give the best chance of achieving *Moksha*. While techniques like yoga and meditation are now common in the West, and practised in isolation, it is in their parent cultures, where the practices are fortified within an overarching belief system and lifestyle, that they have long demonstrated greater innate synergy with conditions conducive to good mental health.

While it may not place at the very summit of the great world religion rankings on mental health, how does the overall record of Western Christianity stack up? Sometimes the need for a clean narrative demands we deal in absolutes, reaching black-or-white judgements. But despite its inarguably abominable diversion into witch hunting, despite Christendom's culpability as a justification for wars down the centuries, and in spite of some unfortunate side effects literal interpretations of doctrine have wrought on medical advancement, it is too easy to conclude that the Western Christian tradition has harmed the human struggle for mental health. Shades of grey are evident. The Bible is ultimately a gospel of hope, compassion and redemption. The New Testament is replete with descriptions of Jesus' demonstrations of love and unconditional forgiveness, from his healing of the blind and sick to the miraculous feeding of the multitudes and ministrations to the poor. It affirms the worth of human beings as bearers of inherent grace, dignity and value. Following this example, the Western Judeo-Christian tradition has made a weighty contribution to the cause of human well-being. Many of Europe's first mental hospitals were Christian institutions, and the foot soldiers of Christian charity have lent their shoulders to charitable causes across the globe. Then, after the witch frenzy was outgrown, the more relaxed strain of Christianity emerging from the Enlightenment fostered the rise of liberal democracy, with its complex but ultimately enriching contribution to the good of humanity. When the chips are counted there is plenty to suggest that the impact of the recent Western rebalance, away from faith and towards secularism, may have been net negative for our mental health – particularly in circumstances where religion has been replaced only with confusion and dissatisfaction. We need to believe in something.

4

THE ANATOMY OF MELANCHOLY – AN ENLIGHTENMENT

Even as Matthew Hopkins was tearing up the English countryside, burning anyone with the temerity not to drown on cue, the first green shoots of a new age of enlightenment were forcing their way to the surface. If the Classical world saw the emancipation of reason, the period spanning the second half of the seventeenth and the eighteenth century witnessed its reawakening. The writings of many ancient Greek and Roman philosophers enjoyed a renaissance of popularity in this era, like friendly whispers carried across an impossible ocean of time to the ears of a world once more ready to hear them. The works of Galileo, Copernicus and Francis Bacon challenged Christianity's philosophical dominion with a starburst of fresh ideas, and the medicos of the age too picked up from where Hippocrates and Galen had left off, questioning religious orthodoxy with a reinvigorated spirit of scientific zeal.

Renaissance Theories of Mental Health

Though belief in supernatural explanations for mental ill health remained popular, alternative naturalistic theories resurfaced to reclaim their place beside them. In 1621 Robert Burton, an Oxford academic, published his encyclopaedic *Anatomy of Melancholy* – an exploration of human nature and an attempt to catalogue mental ill health on an epic scale. Burton made working and reworking the book his life's mission and pursued it unceasingly, using the task as his method for staving off his own psychological issues. 'I write of melancholy, by being busy to avoid melancholy,' he wrote, adding that there is 'no better cure' for mental disturbance than keeping busy.

The 'melancholy' of the title is characteristic of Burton's respect for Classical constructs of mental pathology, but though Burton revives old terminology and revisits ancient conditions, he adds new ones in spades. The first section of his work is a long exposition of many 'common melancholies', while the second deals with their cures. Burton doesn't limit attention to the extreme forms of mental ill health – conditions producing behaviours that inevitably catch society's attention – but writes chiefly about the widespread but often subtle problems that can affect anyone, the mild to moderate issues occurring with such frequency today as to raise the question of whether we are in the grip of a modern epidemic. In a commentary of nearly a thousand pages, Burton also takes on the eternal problem of knowing where lines ought to be drawn in the act of diagnosis, probing the elusive divide between human nature and mental illness:

Melancholy, the subject of our present discourse, is either in disposition or in habit. In disposition, is that transitory Melancholy which goes and comes upon every small occasion of sorrow, need, sickness, trouble, fear, grief, passion, or perturbation of the mind, any manner of care, discontent, or thought, which causes anguish, dulness, heaviness and vexation of spirit, any ways opposite to pleasure, mirth, joy, delight, causing forwardness in us, or a dislike. In which equivocal and improper sense, we call him melancholy, that is dull, sad, sour, lumpish, ill-disposed, solitary, any way moved, or displeased. And from these melancholy dispositions no man living is free, no Stoic, none so wise, none so happy, none so patient, so generous, so godly, so divine, that can vindicate himself; so well-composed, but more or less, some time or other, he feels the smart of it. Melancholy in this sense is the character of Mortality ... This Melancholy of which we are to treat, is a habit, a serious ailment, a settled humour, as Aurelianus and others call it, not errant, but fixed: and as it was long increasing, so, now being (pleasant or painful) grown to a habit, it will hardly be removed.[1]

This demarcation between the normal, emotional response to life's tribulations on the one hand and the problematic state that arises when emotional indispositions become rooted, rather than passing, on the other, fits comfortably with modern ideas about the diagnosis threshold. Today, patients seeking therapy in the immediate aftermath of bereavement or other traumatic experience are often advised to wait a period and see how things develop before starting treatment, in recognition of the time naturally required to overcome adversity as part of a normal process.

Burton backs both horses in the natural-versus-supernatural causality debate and *Anatomy of Melancholy* runs the full gamut of disciplines to illuminate its subject matter, drawing on physiology, philosophy, theology, astronomy and demonology, and listing everything from possession to poverty to heartache among the triggers for the many manifestations of mental illness he describes. Despite giving credence to the possibility of supernatural causes, Burton also points to the Classical physicians with reverence, aspiring to the mantle of being a student of scientific, physiological medicine. He invests great importance in environmental and lifestyle determinants of mental health, noting with a humanist's care the differing problems that can develop when religious devotion, romantic love, or similar intense passions go wrong to become preoccupying or obsessive. To illustrate subtly differing diagnoses with familiar reference points Burton draws on characters from Shakespeare, a trait that anticipated Freud. The distinct flavours of melancholy manifesting in men and women are given life through comparison with Hamlet and Ophelia, and *Much Ado About Nothing*'s Benedick and Beatrice typify Burton's conception of 'Love Melancholy', the stresses wrought by fractious romance. The cures Burton suggests for relieving mental disturbance are similarly broad. Prescriptions of bloodletting, fasting, prayer and bizarre exotic potions sit side by side with talking therapy and recommendations of exercise and relaxation – the struggle between religion and science raging through undecided pages. But Burton reserves particular esteem for the therapeutic value of counselling, framing his case through ancient wisdom once again:

> Whosoever then labours of this maladie (melancholy) the best thing in the world, as Seneca therefore adviseth in such a case by all means let him get some trusty friend ... Tully, if a man had gone to heaven, 'seen the beauty of the skies,' stars errant, &c, *insuavis erit* admiration, it will do him no pleasure, except he have somebody to impart what he hath seen. It is the best thing in the world, as Seneca therefore adviseth in such a case, 'to get a trusty friend, to whom we may freely and sincerely pour out our secrets; nothing so delighteth and easeth the mind, as when we have a prepared bosom, to which our secrets may descend, of whose conscience we are assured as our own, whose speech may ease our succourless estate, counsel relieve, mirth expel our mourning'.[2]

Cartesian Dualism

René Descartes, a contemporary of Burton and a polymath famous for contributions to philosophy, mathematics and science, was another turning his formidable gifts to exploring human nature in the seventeenth century. Descartes went further than Burton by entirely rejecting the religious fulcrum of faith over reason; indeed, Descartes rejected all establishment and received wisdom of any sort. Taking upon himself the great task of reconstructing 'truth' from first principles. He once wrote, 'If you would be a real seeker after truth, it is necessary that at least once in your life you doubt, as far as possible, all things.' He meant it. Descartes dedicated years to rebuilding a theoretical framework of everything, of his own construction and from first building blocks, so he could be sure every link in his chain had been tested and proven sound. He gave us 'I think, therefore I am', was acclaimed as the first modern philosopher, and deserves great credit for helping exorcise lingering demons from some aspects of medicine.

But Descartes' conception of 'dualism', his contribution to the mind/body debate, had far less auspicious ramifications – particularly for mental health. The mind/body conundrum has been debated by scholars and philosophers through the ages. Are the mind and body distinct? What is the nature of their relationship? Dualism was not a new response to these questions when Descartes posited it, but the popularity of his articulation has ensured that it is Descartes with whom the idea is now most closely associated. He theorised that there are two types of substance: matter, with the definitive property of being spatially extended; and mind, defined by its capacity for thought. Descartes reasoned it conceivable that the physical body could exist only as a dream or illusion, and it was therefore possible for him to doubt having a body, but by virtue of being self-conscious enough to have the idea, he could not doubt having a mind.

I suppose therefore that all things I see are illusions; I believe that nothing has ever existed of everything my lying memory tells me. I think I have no senses. I believe that body, shape, extension, motion, location are functions. What is there then that can be taken as true? Perhaps only this one thing, that nothing at all is certain.[3]

Descartes became convinced that the body, if it existed at all, and the mind are fundamentally disparate in materiality (and immateriality), with the implication that very different remedies are required when something goes awry with either part. He identified the pineal gland as the site where the incorporeal soul would dock with the otherwise separate human corpus, and thereby be able to engage the physical, mechanical world. Descartes saw further evidence for his conception of mind/body duality in observations of the animal kingdom, where beasts would act and react reflexively but were little more than automatons in his estimation, devoid of conscious self-awareness and the capacity for reason that elevates humans, guided by their divine souls.

Cartesian dualism proved an attractive idea in a time when many were struggling to reconcile their religious faith with the new, apparently contradictory scientific proofs that the likes of Galileo, Copernicus and Bacon were exploring and tentatively offering up into societies still firmly in the grip of Church authority. For those seeking a rationale that could reason them free of these seemingly insuperable conflicts, Cartesian dualism offered a neat sidestep. The nature and origins of the physical human organism might not be consistent with a literal interpretation of the Bible, but it is not the physical body that God is concerned with, but the human soul – a different thing entirely. On this basis neither the religious establishment nor the new men of science had to be shown up as mistaken. They were both fluent, just in different dialects. To the relief of many who wished to be good, God-fearing citizens despite scientific doubts, direct territorial conflict could be avoided. A cake had and eaten.

Among Descartes' contemporaries Dutchman Baruch Spinoza took the opposing view, rejecting the notion of the mind as an otherworldly construct of mysterious, divine properties. He reasoned that the body and mind were intrinsically bound to form the human whole, and should be considered as one organic entity. Just like the body, Spinoza judged the mind to be a part of the natural world, not a product of a distinct spiritual plane. But bereft of the attractions dualism held for those wishing to reconcile faith and science, Spinoza's counter-arguments did not resonate as favourably in the arena of popular opinion. In the grand debate of dualism versus naturalism, the weight of contemporary opinion cleaved decisively to Descartes. It was a stroke of catastrophe for the cause of mental health – the idea of a mind/body fault line endured for centuries, reinforcing a trajectory that saw medical science concentrate on physical pathology, and the mind and mental disorders abandoned to the compass of the Church. Despite the fact that Descartes himself never advocated these consequences as an axiomatic corollary of his theories, this demarcation was nevertheless a possibility they opened up. Scientific medical enquiry had been legitimised to coexist harmoniously alongside the religious orthodoxy, providing always that activities were restricted to the mechanical, corporeal aspects of human health, and did not trespass into the realm of the immortal soul. The tanks of medicine were not to be parked on the Church's lawn. In consequence, medical attention to the field of mental illness was greatly impoverished relative to endeavours in physical medicine, which received both its green light and head start.

The impacts of this divergence between the physical and the psychological ripple today. According to a 2015 report by the King's Fund, just 11 per cent of the NHS budget is spent on mental health care, despite mental health issues making up 23 per cent of the total 'burden of disease'.[4] Our comparatively underfunded NHS psychological therapy services are also too often siloed, catering only to immediate need, detached from the work of peers in physical health services, and without even exchange of basic patient information that might otherwise facilitate more joined-up care. Our present system is a product of a long inheritance of Cartesian instincts, baked in down many generations. It may provide some short-term comfort, but it is not necessarily the best model for achieving the sustained, holistic outcomes that co-located physical and mental healthcare practitioners acting in concert might deliver.

Mental Health in Literature

Renaissance literature likewise reflects the tension between religion and burgeoning science that defined attitudes towards mental health in the period. The Renaissance was bookended by two great theological works, both among the most influential of all time. Dante Alighieri's epic *Divine Comedy*, completed in 1320, describes Dante's journey through Hell, Purgatory and Heaven, accompanied by Virgil, the great Roman poet. It is soaked in biblical themes. *Paradise Lost*, written by John Milton and published three and a half centuries later in 1667, at the opposite extreme of the Renaissance, is equally fixated on religious tropes. Its epic, dual-arc narrative follows the fall of Satan and the fall of man, retelling Adam and Eve's expulsion from paradise in a reminder of the perils of eating from the tree of knowledge. Both texts centre on themes of sin and salvation, and the idea that mankind's troubles begin and end with questions of faith. There is plenty of mental suffering, but invariably of supernatural agency, or else brought upon mankind by its own breaches of divine law. Abandon hope, ye who enter here.[5]

But as in Classical times, religious paradigms of human psychology were no longer unquestioningly accepted as being the only truth, and more sophisticated renderings of the human condition were also finding acclaim. In between the publication of the *Divine Comedy* and *Paradise Lost*, Miguel de Cervantes framed his description of the madness of the titular character in his *Don Quixote* in the eternal context of the perceptions that attach to someone whose behaviour is out of step with the society they inhabit. Obsessed by outdated notions of chivalric behaviour, the quixotic hero's tilting at windmills, believing them to be giants, is now almost exactly synonymous with baying at the moon – the hopeless act of a deranged soul in the grip of overwhelming internal turmoil. Shakespeare gave us tragic heroes Lear and Othello, whose torments are wholly rooted in interpersonal relationships and reminiscent of the anguishes suffered by Oedipus. Both protagonists are distracted to the point of madness as events swirl around them, Lear agonising over his betrayal by his daughters and Othello wrestling anxious jealousies provoked by Iago's scheming. The plays focus on character as much as dramatic events, with elegant soliloquies illuminating for the audience the inner torment of their heroes. Perhaps Shakespeare's crowning account of human frailty, and the slippery descent into madness, is found in *Hamlet*. Having been visited by the ghost of his father, who declares Hamlet's uncle Claudius his murderer and usurper, the Prince of Denmark affects an 'Antic disposition' – the symptoms of madness – as cover for his revenge. But Hamlet quickly becomes despairing and delusional for real, as he vacillates between believing and disbelieving the reality of his father's ghost. In art, life imitates pretence, as Hamlet lapses into actual obsessive madness, mistakenly murders the father of his love, Ophelia, and sparks a chain of events leading to his own death. What a piece of work humanity is.[6]

Thus the tussle for supremacy raging at the macro level between faith and science, and between natural and supernatural explanations for mental ill health, is visible in concentrate through the literature of the period. Also writing at the time, though his work was only published posthumously, was Samuel Pepys. Centuries before post-traumatic stress disorder was understood, the great diarist recorded how the emotional reaction to traumatic events can swell like a rising tide in their aftermath, with his entries on the Great Fire of London:

I rode down to the waterside ... and there saw a lamentable fire ... Everybody endeavouring to remove their goods, and flinging into the river or bringing them into lighters that lay off; poor people staying in their houses as long as till the very fire touched them, and then running into boats, or clambering from one pair of stairs by the waterside to another. And among other things, the poor pigeons, I perceive, were loth to leave their houses, but hovered about the windows and balconies, till they some of them burned their wings and fell down.[7]

Pepys was later forced by the fire to evacuate his own house, and became involved with attempts to contain it, advising King Charles II to tear down buildings in its path in a vain attempt to halt the spread. The Great Fire famously started in Pudding Lane in September 1666, but Pepys' diary entry of 28 February 1667, months after the immediate shock and adrenaline of events had subsided, recounts his ongoing struggle to process the experience:

It is strange to think how to this very day I cannot sleep a night without great terrors of fire; and this very night I could not sleep till almost 2 in the morning through thoughts of fire.[8]

Another aspect of the relationship between mental health and the arts is the fine line often said to divide insanity from genius. Back in the Graeco-Roman period, a connection between madness, eccentricity and creative genius had been popularised by the likes of Plato, who wrote of the 'divine fury' animating the poet. Roman Stoic Seneca also gave voice to the idea, writing that 'no great genius has existed without a strain of madness', and the etymology of our modern English 'inspiration' derives from the divine act of breathing life into the human form. This association between madness and the spark of artistic creativity survived into the Renaissance and beyond, right up to the first generation of English Romantic poets; among them were Blake and Wordsworth, both prone to severe depression, and Coleridge, also beset by depression and who described himself as occasionally 'irradiated by bursts only of Sunshine' that would give way to moods 'gloomy with clouds, or turbulent with tempests'. A hint of madness was even more intrinsic to the reputation of the second wave – the club of Shelley, Keats and the famously mad, bad Lord Byron, who was dead at thirty-six after an eventful life of extreme action, passions and a brief spell at university spent rooming with a pet bear.

Shelley and Byron were extensively influenced by Goethe's 1774 novel *The Sorrows of Young Werther*, the tale of a hyper-sensitive young man who, tormented by unrequited love, sinks into depression before killing himself with a pistol. The book raised awareness of mental illness, but also made it fashionable, triggering a wave of copycat suicides among young people. Byron thought it a masterpiece but said that it was 'responsible for more deaths than Napoleon himself'. Shelley, who was known as 'Mad Shelley' at Eton, also worshipped the book, and his wife, Mary Shelley, included it in her novel *Frankenstein*, as one of the books read by the monster and which contributes to its education, emotional awakening and eventual murderous rage. The genius of this group is generally acknowledged as having been fired by emotional tumult. Oscar Wilde declared himself convinced that 'all men of genius are insane' while French author Marcel Proust wrote that 'everything great in the world comes from neurotics'. Case study evidence for these views ran deep in the European arts too, with the likes of Rimbaud, Baudelaire and Van Gogh, the latter institutionalised after his notorious ear slicing incident before later taking his own life. Then there was Edvard Munch, who said, 'For as long as I can remember I have suffered from a deep feeling of anxiety which I have tried to express in my art' and whose *Scream* quickly became an iconic portrayal of mental anguish.

We can only speculate whether artists like Munch would have reached the same creative heights had they been free of psychological demons – liberal doses of absinthe and opium were also topping up the genius of many at this time. Nevertheless, the rare quality of their art was popularly taken to be linked with the extreme mental dispositions that helped produce it. A century or two ago, being melancholic or struggling with a 'nervous disorder' could even confer a status approaching fashionable because of this association with a cultured, creative temperament. In this light, the negative stigma that sometimes attaches to mental ill health in the modern age seems more and more a reactionary view, one that some of our ancestors avoided to the great benefit of the arts. Perhaps not coincidentally it was around the time of these great artists that the possibility of useful, diagnostic insights appearing through art also occurred to medics. Italian criminologist and physician Cesare Lombroso pioneered a theory that abnormal levels of absurdity, obscenity and symbolism in paintings betrayed mental instability in the artist – a sentiment that helped many early psychiatrists explain the distasteful excesses they perceived in emergent Expressionist and Surrealist art. Is an inkblot just an inkblot, or a window to the soul? What Lombroso would have made of Banksy we will never know.

Despite the Cartesian red herring, the many luminaries of Renaissance science, philosophy and literature brought about more major advances in attitudes towards mental ill health than had been seen since Classical times, unpicking the supernatural orthodoxy entrenched since the Dark Ages, and disrupting the reductive popular image of the mentally disturbed as mere pitiable unfortunates. Collectively they plotted a course that would blossom into the next remoulding of mental health as a concept. The conditions were set for the birth of a new discipline: psychology.

Psychiatry, Psychology, Psychotherapy and Psychoanalysis

As early as 1690, philosopher John Locke had first construed mental illness as a symptom of dysregulated processing at the point sensory information is received by the mind – essentially, cognitive disturbance. By Cartesian thinking, the notion of a fault with human consciousness was a near contradiction in terms. Since the soul was synonymous with divine reason, any aberrant behaviour *could only* be a malfunction of the mechanical body, not of the mind. To err is, after all, human. Locke's counter-Dualist ideas did not immediately overturn this received wisdom, but they did not altogether go away either. After a slow burn of almost two centuries, German philosopher and physiologist Wilhelm Wundt applied Locke's core ideas within a comprehensive model of mental ill health, predicated on a theory of interconnected feelings, thoughts and behaviours. Published in 1874, Wundt's *Principles of Physiological Psychology* drew together physiology and psychology, and was a runaway success. Wundt went on to establish the world's first psychology laboratory at the University of Leipzig in 1879, offering the first course in scientific psychology. Perhaps without doing full justice to Locke given his contribution, this is often cited as the landmark moment when psychology was first articulated as a distinct scientific discipline, separate from both biological medicine and philosophy. Psychology had previously been regarded as a branch of philosophy, and had been reliant upon feats of abstract reasoning to advance – the kind of philosophising practised by Classical scholars, and of the type Descartes had applied to create truth from first principles in his own head, convincing himself and others besides that he just might be an immense, disembodied consciousness floating in the ether of some *Star Trek* planetoid. Drawing on the natural sciences for his example, Wundt rejected this theoretical approach and pioneered experimental methods of advancing the understanding of psychology, writing:

Psychological inquiries have, up to the most recent times, been undertaken solely in the interest of philosophy; physiology was enabled, by the character of its problems, to advance more quickly towards the application of exact experimental methods. Since, however, the experimental modification of the processes of life, as practised by physiology, oftentimes effects a concomitant change, direct or indirect, in the processes of consciousness – which, as we have seen, form part of vital processes at large, – it is clear that physiology is, in the very nature of the case, qualified to assist psychology on the side of method; thus rendering the same help to psychology that it, itself received from physics. In so far as physiological psychology receives assistance from physiology in the elaboration of experimental methods, it may be termed experimental psychology.[9]

Wundt had created a new discipline, escaping the Cartesian paradigm yet simultaneously managing to maintain a clear divide between the psychiatric and the neurological, with an alternative, naturalistic framework to clear the fogs that had hung like a seemingly impenetrable pall across the boundary between mental illness and medical disorder. Consequently, Wundt is often referred to as one of the fathers of psychology along with Sigmund Freud, who was beginning his own rise to prominence at this time.

Freud was an Austrian neurologist who proposed ideas about the human condition and personality that were radically different even from those of Locke, Wundt and other naturalists. Freud was a co-founder of the International Psychoanalytic Association and developed a number of ideas that underpin the practice of psychotherapy today. His experiences in clinical practice convinced him that early childhood events, and an associated hangover of unconscious, often libidinous impulses, matter most when explaining behaviour. His theories are grounded in the idea that we have both a conscious and an unconscious mind. The conscious is that part occupied with the many details and decisions streaming through our daily awareness, demanding attention so we can navigate our day-to-day interactions; the unconscious, meanwhile, remains aloof but active, processing impulses outside our immediate awareness: the entrenched memories, urges, desires and fears that are latent but influence our behaviour. Freud illuminated his conception of the subconscious mind in his book *The Interpretation of Dreams*:

> The conscious mind may be compared to a fountain playing in the sun and falling back into the great subterranean pool of subconscious from which it rises.[10]

We all intuitively recognise our pet likes, tastes and aversions, and the pattern of choices we typically make in the course of life's routines but can't always rationally explain. Freud awakened us to the unknown psychology lying behind such things: formative experiences, sometimes unpleasant or traumatic, that may have dimmed in the memory but operate imperceptibly, exerting an invisible pull on our behaviour. Freud's later work *The Ego and the Id*, published in 1923, sets out his conception of the mind's structure. Despite the title, Freud identifies three constituent components: the id, the ego and the superego. Each is distinct, influencing our choices in a combination that makes us uniquely 'us' in the blend. According to Freud, the id is part of the unconscious and source of our most primal urges. The ego navigates our day-to-day reality, moderating the urges of the id to keep our behaviour socially appropriate. The superego absorbs, retains and then exerts the influence of life lessons and moral teachings that we acquire in the course of our passing years. Freud believed that mental disturbances often resulted from repressed impulses, and so could be addressed using exploratory dialogue, in other words *talking therapies*, to help patients come to terms with their issues. Because of the importance Freud's theories attributed to the unconscious mind, he placed great value in dreams as 'the royal road to the unconscious', as he described it. For Freud, dreams were full of symbolic importance and an outlet for unconscious feelings that might appear there in metaphorical form. He wrote:

> Obviously one must hold oneself responsible for the evil impulses of one's dreams. In what other way can one deal with them? Unless the content of the dream rightly understood is inspired by alien spirits, it is part of my own being.[11]

For this reason Freud would often use dreams in his clinical practice, inviting patients to recount them as a prelude for his technique of free association, wherein he would take events from dreams as a first link from which to pick up and pursue the chain of thoughts, images and insights connected to them in a patient's mind.

Today, Freud is controversial and his legacy disputed. He theorised that all psychic energy is generated by the libido, heavily correlating human behaviour with instincts for sex, life and death. His 'Oedipus Complex' recalls Sophocles' tragic hero in a theory of children's carnal desire for the opposite sex parent, accompanied by jealousy of the other. He believed that an unconscious wish for death formed an elemental part of the make-up of all human beings, and rationalised self-harm and self-destructive behaviour as manifestations of this 'death drive'. If not full-blown slips, then these ideas must at least qualify as Freudian missteps. They have been derided as speculative, criticised as unprovable and scorned as potentially harmful.

During his formative years Freud spent time in France studying under the eminent neurologist Jean-Martin Charcot, the 'Napoleon of Neurosis', who contributed much to the advancement of neurology but also, controversially, employed hypnotism as a means of diagnosing hysteria. Charcot believed that only people suffering from hysteria were susceptible to hypnotism, and so it offered, therefore, a definitive test for the condition. He trumpeted several of his own patients as evidential case studies, holding court to show them off in well-attended public lectures that adopted the trappings of showbusiness, with live hypnotism as their centrepiece. Charcot's peers were sceptical, seeing in his performances only vulnerable, eager-to-please patients dissembling, consciously or not, in a piece of theatre. They believed Charcot was deceiving himself through a combination of hubris, confirmation bias and ultimately the cold realisation that his reputation was now too far invested for him to turn back. In his *History of Psychiatry*, Edward Shorter describes how medical opinion coalesced to reject

Charcot's ideas, condemning the results of his hypnotisms as the 'artefact of suggestion';[12] in other words, his treatment helped mental health in the same way standing on tiptoes helps make someone taller. Charcot's denunciation widened the scope for critics of psychology to claim that the whole power of this new discipline, all of it and not just the results of eccentrics like Charcot, was really nothing more than a sham. Such allegations long dogged the intangible workings of psychotherapy. Nevertheless, time spent learning from the charismatic Frenchman inspired lasting reverence in Freud, a steadfast disciple of hypnotism's flamboyant guru.

Charcot was not the only divisive figure blundering in darkness while seeking to explain psychological disturbances. Through its infancy, misunderstandings frequently attached themselves to psychotherapy, and those seeking to sanitise the discipline were forced to maintain a constant rearguard effort staving off unwelcome associations with pseudoscientific and even occult ideas that were sometimes conflated with psychology in the public consciousness. Even before Freud had fallen under Charcot's spell, the pet theories of German physicians Franz Mesmer and Franz Joseph Gall had both already come perilously close to fatally undermining the reputation of fledgling psychotherapy. Mesmer's signature belief was that all objects contained a magnetic liquid, shifting with the pull of the moon and planets like the tides.

A responsive influence exists between the heavenly bodies, the earth, and animated bodies. A fluid universally diffused, so continuous as not to admit of a vacuum, incomparably subtle, and naturally susceptible of receiving, propagating, and communicating all motor disturbances, is the means of this influence ... This property of the human body which renders it susceptible of the influence of heavenly bodies, and of the reciprocal action of those which environ it, manifests its analogy with the magnet, and this has decided me to adopt the term of animal magnetism. The action and virtue of animal magnetism, thus characterized, may be communicated to other animate or inanimate bodies. Both of these classes of bodies, however, vary in their susceptibility.[13]

In living beings, Mesmer believed that this fluid determined health according to its flow. He concluded that it was possible for people to harness their 'animal magnetism' to influence others, and considered himself particularly well endowed with the ability. Mesmer opened a clinic in Paris to practise his powers and, like Charcot, held theatrically showy public demonstrations, dressing in long, silken robes and using a magician's wand to direct his concerto of magnetic flows coursing about the bodies of his subjects. Also like Charcot, Mesmer's results depended entirely upon the power of suggestion, but he too was able to earn fleeting acclaim by seemingly spinning straw into gold with a maestro's flourish. But a major controversy was sparked when Mesmer's contemporaries, made uneasy by his habit of spending long hours alone with hypnotised female patients, denounced him as a fraud.

Gall was only nine when his theory of phrenology began to take shape in 1767. The germ of the idea arrived when Gall observed apparent correlations between certain physical characteristics common to a group of his classmates, and other attributes they also shared. His initial observation was that bulging eyes often came paired with an extraordinary facility for memory, something Gall accounted for by reasoning that his schoolmates' eyes were being forced outwards by their brains' exceptionally large frontal lobes – a sure indication, in his reckoning, of these lobes being unusually engorged with memories. On the strength of this Gall considered that he had isolated the locus of memory storage within the brain, and from these beginnings crystallised a full-blown theory mapping twenty-seven distinct faculties and dispositions of temperament with the twinned, narrowly localised regions of the brain that he believed was regulating each one. For him, this map was the key to understanding psychology, and an encoded inevitability driving all human behaviour:

Whoever would not remain in complete ignorance of the resources which cause him to act; whoever would seize, at a single philosophical glance, the nature of man and animals, and their relations to external objects; whoever would establish, on the intellectual and moral functions, a solid doctrine of mental diseases, of the general and governing influence of the brain in the states of health and disease, should know, that it is indispensable, that the study of the organization of the brain should march side by side with that of its functions.[14]

Gall amassed a huge collection of human skulls to help expand his theory. He had specimens that had belonged to people from professions of all kinds, and many from people who, in life, had been considered lunatics and criminals. Always Gall was looking for commonality: the unique lumps, bumps or other clues that would help him pin a tell-tale physical sign to a paired predisposition for a given personality trait, profession, skill or vice. Although Gall's work purported to have a sound basis in science, those studying his work found themselves unable to replicate his correlations. They did uncover huge leaps of inference and assumption amounting to guesswork in Gall's reasoning, leaps that had been necessary to overcome gaps in his logic chain. Perhaps people with bulging eyes are just people with bulging eyes? Phrenology offered a purely biomedical construction of all mental health, ultimately boiling down to the old idea that you *can* judge a book by its cover – but by this time Shakespeare had already proclaimed that 'there's no art to find the mind's construction in the face',[15] and Gall's contemporaries eventually agreed, finding the evidence for phrenology's counterclaims underwhelming beneath the glare of peer scrutiny.

The ideas of Charcot, Mesmer and Gall, though ultimately rejected, still exacted a reputational toll on the image of psychology. A purification was required, and succeeding generations of academic clinicians – luminaries like German psychiatrist Emil Kraepelin, and his colleague Alois Alzheimer, the immortally synonymous specialist in senile dementia – delivered one. They did so by following Wundt's example of applying to psychology the same uncompromising methodologies, statistical techniques and standards of evidential proof that were, and remain, the bedrock of mainstream science, helping liberate the discipline from the unscientific pilot fish ideas bunching around it. In the latter nineteenth century a vibrant international community blossomed, shining the light of scientific rigor into every dark corner of psychology, without bias, fear or favour. By the turn of the twentieth century a ripening psychology movement could claim to have won establishment – indeed nearly universal – esteem as a legitimate field of medicine. It was on these secure foundations that the likes of Freud and Carl Jung, Freud's own protégé, rose to become heralded as visionaries, offering people a fresh window into their innermost souls. The psychoanalyst's canon of work, particularly Freud's concept of the unconscious mind and his surety that talking about mental health problems helps to overcome them, revolutionised how we see mental health.

In the context of considering whether we are experiencing a modern crunch of mental ill health, all this had the pivotal impact of reframing psychological disturbance as something immeasurably more diffuse than the traditional view of it, which had been largely concerned with those labelled 'mad' because of extreme symptoms. Mental ill health was no longer just 'the other'; ordinary people could, probably would, have flare ups of unconscious disturbance from time to time too. Repression and adjustment issues had the potential to manifest in anyone. We all need help sometimes, and new methods were being found to provide it. In this context it is easy to see why many regarded Freud with reverence for overhauling outdated theories of mental health and kicking psychotherapy into something resembling modern practice for the first time. If the package was drawn together with a fanciful bow, that is scant justification for the polemic with which he is sometimes now decried. Following on from Freud's own contributions, his successors took eagerly to the task of sanding the rough edges from his ideas to render their aesthetics all the more finely formed. Carl Jung in particular absorbed his mentor's philosophy like an especially precocious sponge before judging it insufficiently well-tuned, and offering the world a divergent, less libidinously orientated model of analytical psychology. This Jung presented in his seminal work *Psychology of the Unconscious*, published in 1912. It was hugely acclaimed, synthesising and sanitising the best of Freudian thinking while shedding much of the controversy. Then behaviourism, a school that sought to explain human nature through stimuli and conditioning, flourished close on the heels of psychoanalysis, helping counterbalance its introspective, occasionally ivory-tower theorising and refreshing focus on the pragmatic task of working out how best to provide practical, real-world help for people when mental health problems manifested.

Weighed in the balance, the prognosis for humanity's understanding of mental health had improved markedly. The Renaissance delivered the first meaningful breakthroughs in centuries, and even the more outré theories that followed, though subsequently embarrassed by the test of time, at least contributed to the constructive spirit of debate let loose in the period. Reanimated renaissance science had cleared the way for the early psychoanalysts, and in their slipstream a new, more tolerant and inclusive recognition of mental ill health emerged, fostering the understanding that it could affect anyone. In the early twentieth century, academic psychology was energised and the future looked bright; finally light had appeared at the end of mental ill health's long, dark tunnel. But was it really daylight? Or a great big train hurtling towards the coming generations?[16]

5

DAGGERS OF THE MIND – MENTAL HEALTH IN WARTIME

If the pale horse of Disease is indeed mankind's most menacing companion, the bloodied, red horse of War is surely charging close behind. Human history *is* the history of warfare, a long chain of martial conflicts showcasing man's inhumanity to man (for it is much more seldom women who have succumbed to warlike impulses). No corner of the globe is exempt, no civilisation untouched. All wars are tragic, some cataclysmic and after each one the survivors clamour, 'Never again!' and 'We must learn the lessons!' Despite these old refrains, some perspectives are too broad for a single lifetime to absorb and some horrors too potent to grasp as they recede into the fog of time. Books teach us the academic details of past wars – the dates, the victors and the vanquished – but they cannot bring about a true appreciation of the suffering involved once the events they describe have passed from living memory.

Stories handed down the generations lose potency with each telling, and lessons learned with another's blood are too easily forgotten, while old mistakes are repeated time and again, topping up the accounts of aggregate human misery.

Because the question of whether behaviour is considered normal or abnormal depends on the social context surrounding that behaviour, the extraordinary circumstance of war also blurs the lines of mental health. In the theatres of war, actors become enmeshed in the most extreme situations. People break and values shift; the usual standards that govern and boundary behaviour are redrawn, and even the rule of law may be relaxed in line with the state's ability to enforce it. *In extremis*, when people find themselves pushed to the limits of human endurance, personality itself can transform.

Psychological Warfare

Because wars are so often turning points in the histories of nation states, and decisive to the fortunes of the regimes presiding over them, rulers throughout history have attached cardinal importance to the mentality of the troops relied upon to do the fighting. Napoleon's dictum 'In war, moral power is to physical as three to one' captures an idea that has been understood since ancient times by military leaders alive to the immense value of gaining a psychological edge. In consequence, the historical record is ripe with material on mental health in wartime, and packed with vivid, creative examples of psychological warfare. Equally, many terms that have passed into common and medical usage as psychological nomenclature have their origins on the battlefield, where the first observations of a raft of disorders were made by physicians attached to military units – 'siege mentality', 'shell shock' and 'nostalgia' among them.

In the fifth century BCE the Chinese military strategist Sun Tzu produced the much revered *Art of War*, a military treatise that devotes as much importance to battles fought in the mind as it does practical stratagems for managing tactics, supply and terrain in the field. Sun Tzu cites togetherness rather than size as the proper measure of an army's strength, and advocates the value of rigorous mental preparations:

> If you know the enemy and know yourself, you need not fear the result of a hundred battles. If you know yourself but not the enemy, for every victory gained you will also suffer a defeat. If you know neither the enemy nor yourself, you will succumb in every battle.[1]

Ostensibly this passage refers to preparation and tactics, but its wisdom also speaks to self-knowledge, self-possession and confidence. The great importance Sun Tzu attaches to psychology distinguishes *The Art of War* from other early military classics. For him, the critical determinant of a battle's outcome was not the physical struggle, if things ever got to that, but rather the effort to deceive the enemy into incorrectly weighing the military calculus when deciding how to fight – or whether to fight at all. After all, as he wrote, 'The supreme art of war is to subdue the enemy without fighting.'

One method of gaining the victory without battle was to confront the enemy with a display of ferocity so intimidating that their appetite for conflict would be undermined. In what must have been a particularly shocking expression of this tactic, a favourite ploy of Goujian, a fifth-century BCE Chinese ruler, was to order the front line of his troops to cut their own throats before a battle. This horrific spectacle must have left any adversary in no doubt that it was an extraordinary opponent they were about to fight – if they still had the stomach to do so. Around the same time, but on a different continent, a more subtle but equally effective example of psychological warfare was provided by Persian emperor Cambyses II in his campaign against Egypt. The conflict was kindled after Cambyses requested the hand of Egyptian pharaoh Amasis II's daughter in marriage and was offered only the daughter of the previous pharaoh in reply. Deciding that this slight must not pass ignored, Cambyses himself led the subsequent Persian invasion of Egypt. Aware of the reverence Egyptian culture invested in cats, he had feline motifs emblazoned across his soldiers' livery ahead of the fighting. Live cats were even transported along with his troops and distributed amid their lines to further intimidate and inhibit their Egyptian opponents whenever they were engaged. The subsequent Battle of Pelusium, fought in 525 BCE, ended in victory for Cambyses and a complete rout of the Egyptians; Herodotus records the Egyptian losses as being some seven times those suffered by their Persian adversaries, although there is a disturbing lack of clarity on the cats' fates in his reckonings.

Perhaps the most famous of all examples of psychological warfare was the signature tactic of Vlad Tepes, or Vlad the Impaler, whose popular moniker attests to the value he placed on weakening his enemies with fear before attacking them. When the Ottoman Empire invaded his home territory of Wallachia in 1462, Vlad adopted a scorched earth policy in retreat, poisoning wells and torching crops in front of Sultan Mehmed's advancing army. Meanwhile, Vlad had his own troops harass the Ottoman camps after nightfall, seeking to weaken their resolve with guerrilla raids. Finally reaching Vlad's capital at Târgoviște after weeks of arduous marching under the threat of these attacks, the Ottomans were amazed to discover the gates undefended and no resisting army marshalled to meet them. Instead they were met by the hideous sight of a vast human forest of men, women and children impaled on stakes and rotting outside of the capital. The Greek historian Chalkokondyles estimated 20,000 bodies in all, covering an area of seven acres. After witnessing this, and with nothing resembling a conventional standing army left to fight against, Mehmed is said to have acknowledged the diabolical nature of his adversary and immediately turned his army for home.

A show of strength has long been regarded as critical in conflict; establishing psychological superiority is vital. The most astute generals would not give an inch of compromise in pursuit of this objective. In the run-up to the American War of Independence, as Britain sought to avoid all-out war with a negotiated settlement, letters outlining their proposals were addressed to 'Mister Washington Esquire' – the British refusing to recognise Washington as a real general at the head of a legitimate army. Washington sent them all back unopened. He dug his heels in over the little details, signalling the same unbending determination which would characterise his leadership of the subsequent battles too, until after seven years of war Washington was finally able to drive the British from the United States, securing its status as a free and independent nation.

A different kind of slow terror arises when warfare turns to stalemate and then siege. In such a situation the defensive forces, and any civilians remaining within the confines of the besieged city's walls, were faced with a particularly unattractive set of potential outcomes. The siege might result in their city's fall, bringing the enslavement or murder of its people; if defences held, on the other hand, the siege would perhaps end only after their slow starvation. Those besieged in this way would be forced to endure a unique form of helpless uncertainty while praying for a miracle of deliverance as reserves of supplies dropped ever lower. Some sieges were torturously protracted. In the course of the Punic Wars the Roman siege of Carthage lasted a full three years before succeeding, with the city then razed to the ground and its entire population killed or sold into slavery. Through its decline, the Roman Empire itself endured a series of sieges at the hands of the Barbarians, Goths and Huns as province after province was attacked. Imagine the terror that must have resulted from the sight of Attila, scourge of God, at a city's gates, bent on an accelerated programme of genocide. Attila's infamy spread rapidly as city after city was sacked, their populations put to death in the wake of his marauding depredations as horrific examples of the perils of resisting the Hun. Into modern history too, the major seats of power have had to endure the ravages and psychological torments of siege warfare. Among the most bloody and famous examples are Tenochtitlan, where the Aztec civilisation fell to the Spanish; Sevastopol, where the Russians dug in against a combined force of Turks, French and British; Leningrad in the course of the Second World War in the face of the Nazi onslaught; and Vienna, which endured Ottoman sieges in 1529 and again in 1683 before John Sobieski's winged hussars relieved the beleaguered, traumatised inhabitants.

Little wonder the phrase 'siege mentality' has entered our language and today describes the shifted plane of thought that can arise when we are assailed by threats. It is now often used in reference to paranoia, a mindset where possibly imaginary threats are perceived and everything and everyone is presumed to be a threat, producing undue defensiveness. (Although 'undue' is not a term that could be legitimately employed to those experiencing it in the live theatre of war – just because you're paranoid doesn't mean the invader won't kill you if your defences are breached.) When the Covid-19 outbreak forced nations throughout the world into lockdown, modern communities received some slight insight into the psychological stresses involved as millions were forced to hunker down in the shadow of an uncertain threat.

In the concentrated state of a siege mentality, surprising ingenuity and desperate tactics can often result. In medieval times the defenders of besieged cities would sometimes catapult food into attacker encampments, demonstrating to their enemies the plentiful reserves they possessed. Local folklore, possibly apocryphal, holds that the city of Carcassonne in southern France was named in honour of an occasion when Lady Carcas, an eminent former citizen, employed this tactic after her city came under siege from Charlemagne's Frankish forces in the eighth century. After five long years of stalemate, Carcassonne's supplies were running perilously low when Lady Carcas hit upon the idea of fattening up a pig and catapulting it over the city walls into the Frankish encampment. As she had hoped, this convinced the Franks that Carcassonne had enough provisions to hold out indefinitely, and they promptly withdrew. If true, this story represents a brilliant example of psychological warfare employed in a context of siege mentality – a desperately bizarre tactic, perhaps, but one that brought the standoff to a happy conclusion for the citizens of Carcassonne. Except, of course, for the pig, who may have found occasion to reflect on the irony of his airborne situation, perhaps even on the nobility of sacrifice, while whistling through the clouds in the direction of the Frankish forces.

Shell Shock and Post-traumatic Stress Disorder

Nostalgia is another term describing a psychological state with roots in military history. It was coined by eighteenth-century Swiss physician Johannes Hofer, who applied it to the strange, depressed condition he noticed afflicting troops stationed away from home on long tours of duty. In 1761, Hofer's Austrian contemporary Josef Auenbrugger developed the observations of this mystery malaise in his

Inventum Novum, providing a fuller description of the mental traumas plaguing stricken soldiers:

> When young men who are still growing are forced to enter military service and thus lose all hope of returning safe and sound to their beloved homeland, they become sad, taciturn, listless, solitary, musing, full of sighs and moans. Finally, they cease to pay attention and become indifferent to everything which the maintenance of life requires of them. This disease is called nostalgia. Neither medicaments, nor arguments, nor promises, nor threats of punishment are able to produce any improvement.[2]

Today the term 'nostalgia' might evoke images of someone experiencing sad, sepia-tinted reminiscences or homesickness, but back when the likes of Auenbrugger were trying to rationalise the psychological conditions accompanying war, the definition overlapped with symptoms that would now be associated with post-traumatic stress disorder, or PTSD. The early conception of nostalgia was very broad, and under this broad definition the blood-soaked battles of the American Civil War led to it becoming the second most common diagnosis made by Union doctors in the 1860s.[3] During the Civil War the symptoms that Hofer and Auenbrugger had clustered together as nostalgia were also referred to variously as 'exhausted heart' and 'soldier's heart' as American physicians too struggled to pin down the particular anguish afflicting overwrought soldiers. As well as their yearning for home, the symptoms recorded among Civil War combatants and attributed to this catch-all condition included tremors, self-harm, palpitations and even catatonic paralysis. Author Ambrose Bierce fought on the Union side in the conflict and took part in the Battle of Shiloh, where 23,000 men lost their lives amid fierce fighting in April 1862. Many years after the war Bierce wrote that he was still traumatised by his experiences there, plagued by flashbacks of dying men. Similarly, future United States President James Garfield was forever changed by the Civil War. Garfield had served as a major general and saw action, and death, at Middle Creek and Chickamauga as well as Shiloh. Nineteenth-century author William Dean Howells described the powerful impact these experiences had on the future president:

> At the sight of these dead men whom other men had killed, something went out of him, the habit of a lifetime, that never came back again: the sense of the sacredness of life and the impossibility of destroying it.[4]

Today, both Garfield and Bierce might be speedily diagnosed with post-traumatic stress disorder. But PTSD is a condition that had a long wait for recognition, its journey particularly hindered by what is known as the stigma impediment, something which runs through the history of mental health like a toxic watermark. Amid the macho culture of the military, trauma sustained on the battlefield was often suppressed for fear of it being taken as cowardice. This held back both our understanding of PTSD and the development of effective treatments for relieving it, and it is impossible to estimate the vast numbers of combatants who must have suffered in silence as a result of feeling unable to ask for help.

This silent suffering was an avoidable tragedy; the potential damage wrought on the psyche by trauma, not just that resulting from experiences on the battlefield but any major damage, is something that had long been known. It can be detected in contemporary medicine and literature, and also to some degree in the popular understanding. Shakespeare gifted the world a painfully exquisite account of PTSD through his portrayal of the mental anguish of Macbeth as the Thane of Cawdor grapples with his 'dagger of the mind' having murdered Duncan. In the days before broadcast and social media, it is hard to imagine how a description of mental trauma could have reached a greater audience than through the Bard. But medical and state recognition of PTSD would not arrive for another four centuries, and later still came due compassion and care for its sufferers. It was 1980 before the American Psychiatric Association added post-traumatic stress disorder to its *Diagnostic and Statistical Manual of Mental Disorders*, but it was during the First World War that the events that would ultimately result in this official classification had begun to gather irresistible momentum. The sheer number of Great War combatants reporting symptoms like those experienced by Garfield and Bierce meant that the psychological aftereffects of battle trauma could no longer be ignored. It accelerated the process of finding a name for their pain, and that name, as bestowed in the early 1900s, was 'shell shock'.

The term shell shock first reached public consciousness in 1917 when Charles Myers, a captain in the Royal

Medical Corps and Director of the Cambridge Psychological Laboratory, wrote a paper on the condition for *The Lancet*. Myers' piece was the first appearance of the term in medical literature. Its victims were described as suffering from symptoms including withdrawal, trauma and an inability to sleep or eat. More seriously in the eyes of the top brass, they were also rendered incapable of fighting, with unedifying consequences as battle trauma was often conflated with cowardice. The name shell shock was chosen because its symptoms were initially supposed to be the direct result of a soldier getting caught close to an exploding shell, sufficiently distant to avoid immediate obliteration or even to escape any obvious, outward damage but within a blast zone thought to trigger the psychological disturbances observed. Some medics theorised that subtle damage to the nerves might accrue in an attritional fashion through prolonged exposure to the protracted, heavy bombardments that characterised much of the Great War. The scale of the problem was massive, with huge numbers of soldiers returning from the trenches mute, blind, deafened or paralysed. Many were haunted by visions of the horrors they had witnessed in combat long after the battles were over. Soldier and war poet Siegfried Sassoon offered first-hand testimony of the impacts of shell shock in his 1917 poem 'Survivors', describing the 'broken' condition of returnee soldiers left repairing shattered lives and dreaming dreams that 'drip with murder'.[5]

Sassoon served on the Western Front and distinguished himself by his bravery, having been credited with the single-handed capture of a German trench after scattering its occupants with a grenade in an action that won him the Military Cross in 1916. 'Survivors' was written a year later while Sassoon was himself recovering from shell shock at Edinburgh's Craiglockhart Hospital, and having grown cynical about what he considered the exploitation of humble soldiers by remote sabre rattlers sending them to their deaths too casually. Along with his friend and fellow war poet Wilfred Owen, another shell shock sufferer, Sassoon produced work that reached a wide audience, helping influence public opinion on the war and the plight of veteran combatants struggling with its aftermath. While it has been suggested that his sojourn at Craiglockhart might have owed as much to War Office desires to discredit and remove a troublesome critic from the front lines as it did to genuine medical needs, Sassoon was undoubtedly deeply traumatised by his experiences in the trenches.

Owen, who had voluntarily returned to the fighting after his own treatment, never made it back again from the killing zones of France, progressing to his 'distant rest'[6] having been killed in action just a week before Armistice Day. But Sassoon was one among the legions of ravaged troops left adjusting to much changed lives back in Britain shortly thereafter, and medics at home, in Craiglockhart and elsewhere, were just as mystified as their field-based colleagues had been when it came to understanding the strange malaise afflicting so many among their number. As for those shell shock victims whose symptoms were misattributed to some fault of character, many found themselves facing formal charges of cowardice or desertion. Some of those convicted were even condemned to death –

the ultimate injury piled on top of insult. But by the end of the war more than 80,000 people suffering with shell shock had passed through British Army medical facilities, and more than twenty hospitals throughout the UK were dedicated to managing the wave of sufferers,[7] some having been repurposed expressly towards this end. This was fallout on a scale so monumental it could no longer be written off as cowardice. The effects lingered long afterwards, even if society increasingly wished to move on from the war. One prominent figure who did not turn his back on these men was Winston Churchill. Drawing attention to their plight in a speech on behalf of 'mentally disabled ex-servicemen' at Mansion House in 1934, he spoke of how 'shell shock and the other strange horrors of Armageddon' had given rise to a 'loss of hope' in them, beneath 'inky waters of despair'. These hollowed-out legions finally forced a pained acknowledgment from the military and political authorities that something of real substance and medical legitimacy was happening. Though it came far too late for those traumatised veterans already shot as deserters, the resulting attention did prove the first step to the official recognition of PTSD that arrived so belatedly in 1980.

The Second World War

By the middle of the twentieth century, humanity had progressed in fitful steps to its most recent martial cataclysm: the Second World War. Even as survivors of the previous conflict, like Sassoon, looked on with sorrowful eyes, a new generation was pushed blindly after them. The Nazi blitzkrieg exploded across Europe and muscled through country after country in rapid succession, limitrophe territories collapsing like dominoes before the advancing panzers. In their wake, the tragedies of war were visited on another generation of Europeans. Countless lives, each one of immeasurable value, were thrown away. The Second World War would stretch six years and it was only when it neared its end, as the Allies entered the camps at Dachau, Auschwitz and Bergen-Belsen on the heels of their retreating enemy, that the full human horror of the conflict was revealed. The Nazi contribution to the history of mental health, as with so many things, was dreadful. There were many labels that were dangerous to have attached to your name if you were living under the authority of Nazi-occupied Europe, and mentally ill was one such. The Nazis are estimated to have slaughtered at least 220,000 people because they were deemed mentally defective.[8] This tally included huge numbers with a diagnosis of schizophrenia, as Hitler's regime attempted the complete eradication of the condition within the boundaries of the Reich. Beyond these killings, many more mentally unwell people were forcibly sterilised, furthering the grotesque Nazi programme of eugenics that also targeted for destruction Jews, Slavs, Roma, homosexuals and the physically disabled. These were the people the Nazis considered *Lebensunwertes Leben* – lives unworthy of life.

On the opposing side of this titanic struggle, the endurance of the Allies was being tested to its limits. People in occupied Europe suffered terribly under the Nazi yoke and in Britain, the last bastion of resistance, the ever-present threat of invasion inflicted colossal stress upon the national psyche. With all Europe seemingly prone before the Nazi advance it was the British Prime Minister, Winston Churchill, to whom fate entrusted the future of the continent, and it was Churchill who rose to the supreme occasion to earn his place among the great wartime leaders. With unswerving certainty and inspirational words Churchill breathed fortitude into Allied resistance, maintaining the light of hope in Europe during the continent's darkest hour. The people responded, sustaining their steadfast efforts and, in Britain, sustaining too the famed 'stiff upper lip' throughout the seemingly hopeless days of the early 1940s before slowly, and at terrible cost, the tide of war began to turn in the Allies' favour.

Churchill's was a life of extraordinary accomplishment and crushing responsibility. It was an exacting burden, and he endured a long personal struggle with depression. Even before the First World War Churchill experienced acute episodes of his symptoms, confiding in his doctor,

> For two or three years, the light faded from the picture. I did my work. I sat in the House of Commons. But a black depression settled on me.[9]

This 'black dog' of depression, as Churchill whimsically called it, was a lifelong companion. Another quote reveals how closely to the surface it bubbled, in spite of his granite public image:

> I don't like standing near the edge of a platform when an express train is passing through. I like to stand back and,

if possible, get a pillar between me and the train. I don't like to stand by the side of a ship and look down into the water. A second's action would end everything. A few drops of desperation.[10]

Churchill is not alone among the iconic war leaders in his mental struggles. Hugely speculative as such retrospective diagnosis must be, commentators have variously attached labels of bipolar, manic depressive, narcissistic and psychopathic to contemporary dictators Hitler and Stalin, and going back further to Napoleon too. Certainly all exhibited seemingly inhuman emotional detachment, great capacity for energetic action, a ruthless disposition and a robust vein of fierce ambition running front and centre through their characters. In Churchill's case, however, his awareness of his own vulnerability to depression and suicidal thoughts may have informed the primary importance he attached to sustaining the morale and hopes of the British populace, the objective he pursued most famously through his speeches.

By the end of the Second World War, in no small part owing to Churchill's grit, the Allies had prevailed. The Reich that was meant to have lasted a thousand years had fallen somewhat short, managing twelve, and humanity has never been better served than by the nations that brought about its destruction. But their peoples had weathered a terrible ordeal. In the midst of the carnage another phrase had been coined, and quickly became synonymous with the British identity: 'Blitz spirit'. As British physical defences, and even the valiant efforts of 'the Few', had failed to halt the Luftwaffe's bombardments of winter 1940 and spring 1941, this spirit had been about the only bulwark left sustaining the people. In these months Nazi bombing raids were a nightly occurrence as the Luftwaffe pursued Hitler's objective of smashing British morale. Buoyed by Churchill, the famous 'stiff upper lip' was the instrument that spurred people through those long, dark days when the war came to British shores and invasion was a real possibility. But what toll did the horrors exact from the survivors? This was a generation that experienced extraordinary conditioning; did it result in mass desensitisation to horrific events? Could this partly explain why the mental health issues of succeeding generations might *feel* like a modern epidemic in comparison, juxtaposed with the experiences of immediate ancestors so inured to the events of war? At the time of the war, much was necessarily made of the cliché image of the English persona as one of quiet resilience, with extreme emotions regarded almost as some congenital defect that ought to be suppressed. So could some inherent hardness of spirit, unique to the Second World War generation, also explain why shell shock features so much more prominently in the narrative about the First World War than the Second?

While the terrors of the Blitz were undoubtedly met with remarkable fortitude, and while the mental scars of war were worn bravely by civilians and military alike, it is not true that widespread psychological consequences were avoided. Despite being most closely associated with the First World War, post-traumatic stress was as much part of the aftermath of the second as it had been the first. But one thing had changed – by the time of the Second World

War, recent experience had taught military authorities to manage things very differently, employing what amounted – from their perspective at least – to a much more skilful handling of wartime 'PR'. Soldiers at the front who suffered a mental disturbance were often quickly sedated to knock them out, then typically described as 'exhausted' – a term deliberately chosen to de-medicalise their condition. It was feared that if shell shock was officially recognised then a great proliferation, as had characterised the First World War, could grow virally by encouraging more and more men to believe they were ill, creating subconscious susceptibility that would further spread the condition. This was an unwelcome prospect for military commanders who did not want to normalise, or even acknowledge shell shock if it risked depleting front-line resources even more. In the absence of reliable data we cannot know for sure, but this 'message management' and deliberate effort to contain events suggests there is no reason to think that prevalence of battle related trauma was any different in the Second World War than it had been in the first. Snippets of anecdotal evidence are available. We know, for example, that US Army General George Patton found two shell shocked soldiers when visiting military hospitals in Sicily in 1943, before promptly slapping both, insisting they were cowards with no legitimate medical complaint at all. But, in contrast to attitudes in the First World War, we know too that public outrage at Patton's actions later forced him into making an apology to the soldiers involved. Attitudes were changing, both among the public and the political and military elite, but certainly shell shock had not gone away.

This is not to diminish the legend of the stiff-upper-lipped British soldier, or the Blitz spirit of the people they fought to defend. Many brave veterans and civilians alike did suppress their wartime trauma, and many must have suffered all the more for having done so. Wartime phrases that seemingly imply emotional coldness, such as airmen's casual references to friends and comrades having 'got the chop' or 'bought it', served, in part at least, as coping mechanisms to help them focus on the terrifyingly risky missions assigned to them, a useful expedient that sustained them through extraordinary times. But admirable self-mastery can carry risks when emotional regulation tips into emotion denial. Today, it is more generally accepted that traumatic events inevitably carry an emotional cost, and that admitting it is no weakness. Working through all this, processing wartime experiences in the collective public consciousness, was an important step on the long journey towards normalising the idea that it is sometimes okay to *not* feel okay, the point where misplaced shame no longer prevents so many people suffering psychological issues from seeking help. Their contribution to this process was just one among the many, many blessings bestowed upon the world by the brave sacrifices of our wartime generation of heroes.

6

ASYLUMS AND AGONY –
INSTITUTIONALISATION AND
EXPERIMENTAL TREATMENTS

I would rather have a bottle in front of me than a frontal lobotomy, as the old joke goes. It is a hard sentiment to dispute. Self-medication by alcohol may not be ideal but it remains infinitely preferable to the prospect of a lobotomy, or many other putative remedies for mental ill health attempted through history. Some were gruesome and personally devastating for those subjected to them, inflicting damage that far outweighed any benefits conferred. Early remedies designed according to a supernatural interpretation of mental ill health were characterised by the violence that might be expected from people believing they were combatting evil spirits rather than treating patients. It is incredible to think that the earliest archaeological evidence of trepanning – boring into the skull for reasons interpreted as medical – dates from about 6,500 BCE, and that some eight thousand years later, with humanity still desperately searching for a means of treating severe mental disturbance, the practice witnessed a resurgence of popularity. Albeit dressed up in a new guise, with faux medical credentials and rebranded as lobotomy for its second coming, it was essentially just trepanation, scraped from the floor of history and shoved back into the oven for a desperate reheating. Its popularity restored, the practice of lobotomy then endured for decades, remaining a commonplace treatment option in the United Kingdom and the United States right up to the mid-twentieth century. Ignorance is not wickedness but can be just as ruinous.

Dangerous Treatments

This revival of the lobotomy as a modern surgical technique began in the late 1800s, the aim of the lobotomist surgeons at this time being merely to quieten the most violently agitated patients, rendering them docile enough to be controlled. There was little serious expectation that the procedure would restore sanity, or improve cognitive functioning, and an operation that resulted in the patient entering a vegetative state would have been deemed a success. The practitioners performing these early lobotomies were still working with only a rudimentary idea of which parts of the brain control what, and their technique was to drill through the skull in the general direction of the nerve fibres connecting the frontal lobe with the rest of the brain. The transorbital lobotomy followed in the twentieth century and involved inserting a pick-shaped instrument into the eye cavity, where it would hook upwards to reach the thin bone separating the eye socket from the frontal lobe. The surgeon would then tap the pick to penetrate both bone and brain with, one hopes, carefully measured force and a better chance of hitting the intended target. Even today, with the benefit of detailed magnetic resonance imaging of the brain, our understanding of the dynamics of neural pathways and complex firings of synapses remains so incomplete that treatment of brain injuries remains soaked in guesswork. Because of the manifest difficulties in accessing a living brain *in situ*, surgery is reserved as a last resort; it is not something a physician would contemplate without urgent necessity. It doesn't take a neurosurgeon to work out that the safest course must be to resist any speculative impulse to cut clumsily into this most delicately balanced of organs – but lobotomy *was* brain surgery, of a crude sort, with terrifyingly uncertain outcomes and prognosis.

When Antonio Moniz carried away the Nobel Prize for Medicine in 1949 for pioneering the prefrontal lobotomy, the award was testimony to the dearth of alternatives available at the time, and the desperation with which the medical establishment received any technique apparently able to calm their most acutely agitated patients. Most lobotomies brought neither comfort to the patient nor cure to the disease, but in the absence of alternatives the procedure grew in popularity, and some well-known people underwent it. Rosemary Kennedy, sister of future President John F. Kennedy, suffered from seizures and extreme, occasionally violent mood swings through childhood. Her parents became concerned by her slow development and apparent mental limitations from a young age. Although it has been unkindly suggested that their impression of these limitations may have been distorted by comparison with her gifted siblings, Kennedy had suffered complications at birth, restricting her oxygen supply and likely causing her stunted developmental path. In 1941 her father Joseph, the Kennedy family patriarch, arranged for Rosemary to receive a prefrontal lobotomy. She was just twenty-three, and a chilling account of the procedure based on an interview with one of the doctors involved is included in Ronald Kessler's 1996 biography of Joseph. It describes Rosemary being asked to recite the Lord's Prayer as the surgeons made their incisions, judging when to stop according to the point at which Rosemary became incoherent.[1] The operation was an abject failure. Her outbursts stopped, but for Rosemary pretty much everything else stopped too. Having formerly lived a social and active life, she was afterwards confined to an institution to live out the rest of her days, unable to speak intelligibly or walk normally. Rosemary endured more than sixty years in this condition before passing away in her eighties.

The Asylums

Another fall-back solution to the problem of managing people deemed too violently disturbed to walk the streets of nineteenth- and early twentieth-century Western society was the asylum. London's Bethlem Royal Hospital, known simply as Bedlam, had come into being far earlier, having been founded as a monastic retreat and refuge for the homeless in 1247 during the reign of Henry III. Following its foundation, Bedlam gradually drifted towards specialising in the care of the insane, a repurposing that was accelerated when Henry VIII's sixteenth-century dissolution of the monasteries meant that the status of secular hospital was suddenly far more expedient than that of monastic retreat. It was Henry who, in 1547, granted the 'custody, order and government' of Bedlam to the City of London, as one of the five royal hospitals re-instituted after the Reformation. In the years since, the happenings within Bedlam's walls have attracted fascination and criticism in not quite equal measure. Opening its gates to the paying public like some grotesque tourist attraction became standard practice at Bedlam, a policy that left the institution vulnerable to accusations of indulging voyeurism. It also earned the notoriety that cemented 'Bedlam' as a byword for chaos. The sight greeting Bedlam's early visitors was certainly not a pretty one, with restraint in irons, bloodletting and dousing patients alternately in hot and cold water among the therapies exhibited for public spectacle. Bedlam's authorities distanced themselves from the unwelcome optics of profiteering from human misery with carefully constructed cover. The real object of Bedlam's open-door policy may have been to swell the coffers, but the official explanation was one of public service; they offered a warning against the perils of vice, sin and impiety, lest the spectator's own life should lead them to Bedlam.

Remarkably, although some private and religiously organised sanatoriums or 'mad houses' sprang up in the intervening years, Bedlam remained England's only public mental institution until the 1800s. Prior to this, responsibility for caring for the mentally disturbed, and particularly the obligation to safeguard society from them, was conventionally considered a domestic obligation resting with immediate family, similar to the assumed duty of parents to control the behaviour of their children. This was consistent with tradition since Classical times. In circumstances where there existed no family able or willing to assume responsibility, the afflicted would typically have been abandoned to the streets to take their chances as beggars, and the greatly foreshortened lifespan likely to result would have been considered an organic, if brutal, mechanism for ridding society of a problem. Even by the turn of the nineteenth century, the great bulk of people suffering serious psychological issues were completely forsaken. Many were left destitute and scratching out a living from day to day, or else languishing in workhouses or in jails; a shortcoming of Georgian society that should perhaps be judged sympathetically, given the symmetry with our own, modern-day prison population.

This landscape changed radically as asylums surged in number through the Victorian era, a growth triggered by events set in motion when Victoria's grandfather George III survived an attempted assassination. The king's would-be assassin, James Hadfield, had fought the French in the name of king and country at the Battle of Tourcoing in 1794, where he suffered repeated blows from a sabre. He was left with head injuries that were both serious and disfiguring, but survived to return to England. Having done so, Hadfield developed a bizarre delusion; he convinced himself that the second coming of Christ would be presaged by his own death, and conceived a spectacular method of bringing it about. In 1800 Hadfield attended a performance at the Drury Lane theatre, and using a concealed pistol took aim at the king in the royal box. Hadfield's shot missed, and he was quickly apprehended and charged with high treason. There can be little doubt that someone so obviously guilty of trying to kill a king, in front of so many witnesses, would have been speedily executed just a century or two before; it is hard to imagine monarchs like Henry VIII or Charles I tolerating any lesser outcome. But two doctors testified that Hadfield's actions were the product of insanity – a direct result of the still obvious head injuries he had suffered in the service of the king – and with this in mind the presiding judge felt compelled to acquit him. In a twist, however, the judge also ruled that though Hadfield lacked the capacity to be truly culpable of the charges against him, he was also evidently too dangerous to remain free, and so should be confined rather than released as would usually have been the outcome when a defendant was found not guilty by reason of insanity. The state had thereby created a new category of people who were not criminals but who could not be left at liberty either, and so also manufactured for itself a major new problem working out what to do with them. The result was the Criminal Lunatics Act of 1800. It sanctioned indefinite detention of criminally insane defendants, and it meant that the state would soon need far more than the single asylum at Bedlam to accommodate people who could no longer be executed, accommodated within the regular prison system or thrown back onto the streets, as would hitherto have been the case.

The subsequent spread of asylums moved at such pace that less than a hundred years later, in the middle of the Victorian era, England boasted more than a hundred mental institutions.[2] Urgency had been injected by the Lunacy Act and accompanying County Asylums Act, both of 1845, which had made it compulsory for every county to build an asylum. The result was a new, nationwide institutional infrastructure, attuned to the fresh requirements of the law. This building programme arranged the structural ducks needed to facilitate mass migration away from communities, prisons and workhouses and into asylums in a neat row, but the predictable result was a grand proliferation of quacks. The popular image of the Victorian asylum and the physicians ruling over them is a forbidding one, and rightly so. Although the numbers entering asylums were climbing fast, far fewer ever left, and once committed to an asylum patients were at the complete mercy of presiding physicians and managers. Early asylums encountered little in the way of independent scrutiny, and at their worst were tyrannical regimes, meting out ghastly treatments in an almost complete vacuum of regulatory oversight. Within their precincts 'therapy' often amounted to little more than lesser forms of torture. Bloodletting and blistering of patients were both commonly employed, and round-the-clock physical restraint with manacles was standard practice. Also popular was the 'Gyrating Chair', an instrument conceived with the intention of shaking its sitter back to equilibrium, but which typically just rendered them unconscious. An account of the violence that characterised the worst excesses of the nineteenth-century asylum system was published by former

Bedlam inmate Urban Metcalf in *The Interior of Bethlem Hospital*:

> Another patient named Harris, for the trifling offence of wanting to remain in his room a little longer one morning than usual, was dragged by Blackburn (a warden), assisted by Allen, the basement keeper, from No. 18, to Blackburn's room, and there beaten by them unmercifully; when he came out his head was streaming with blood, and Allen in his civil way wished him good morning. The case of Morris; this man had some pills to take, which he contrived to secrete in his waistcoat pocket, this Blackburn discovered, and by the assistance of Allen, they got him to his room and there beat him so dreadfully for ten minutes as to leave him totally incapable of moving for some time, Rodbird was looking out to give them notice of the approach of any of the officers; they are three villains. A man by the name of Baccus, nearly eighty years of age, was this summer admitted into the house; one very hot day he had laid down in the green yard, another patient named Lloyd, very much disordered, trod on the middle of his body purposely, this Blackburn the keeper encouraged by laughing, and Lloyd would have repeated it, but something diverted his attention: Baccus is since dead.[3]

These early madhouses, and their ghoulish apparatus, often became the last domicile of unfortunate, unemployed paupers, trapped in the orbit of a bloated asylum system as it grew and grew throughout the nineteenth century. Asylums also served as holding pens for traumatised veterans of the Army or Navy, in the years before the fallout of the First World War, with its epic scale, forced recognition of shell shock upon the medical establishment.

In the early twentieth century, these well-stocked asylums proved convenient testing grounds for a controversial new treatment: electroconvulsive therapy, or ECT. The desperate need to manage the many shell-shocked individuals returning home from the Great War lent great appeal to this new therapy, which was apparently cheap as well as effective. ECT involves sending a current into the brain, creating a surge of electrical activity to bring about a seizure. As of 2020 it remains on the list of treatments recommended by the UK's National Institute for Health and Care Excellence (NICE) for severe cases of depression or mania. But some of the unethical applications ECT has been put to in the past have given the treatment a controversial reputation. Until the late 1960s, in times when homosexuality remained illegal in the United Kingdom, ECT, along with aversion therapy, was forcibly administered in an attempt to 'cure' people of what was then considered an aberrant perversion. It was only in 1973 that the American Psychiatric Association removed homosexuality from its official *Diagnostic and Statistical Manual of Mental Disorders*. Before then, as the treatment of choice for such cases, the reputation of ECT was caught up with the controversy and injustice of treating sexuality as pathology, taking a hammering in the process.

The case of Ernest Hemingway, perhaps the most famous recipient of ECT, also did nothing to further its reputation. In 1918, the eighteen-year-old Hemingway caught the tail end of the First World War and was mortared and seriously injured while serving as an ambulance driver in Italy. Hemingway found himself among the ranks of shell-shocked survivors, and struggled with depression for the rest of his life. Forty years after his wartime experiences, and suffering from increasingly poor physical health, hypertension and paranoia, Hemingway underwent several episodes of ECT in the winter of 1960 and spring of 1961 in the months before his death. It resulted in Hemingway losing much of his memory, and he lamented the results.

> What these shock doctors don't know is about writers and such things as remorse and contrition and what they do to them. Well, what is the sense of ruining my head and erasing my memory, which is my capital, and putting me out of business? It was a brilliant cure, but we lost the patient.[4]

The patient who already considered himself lost was soon to be gone in every sense. Hemingway shot himself at his home in Idaho in July 1961.

The negative reputation of techniques like ECT and lobotomy combined with the already bleak popular image of the institutions in which they were practised to earn asylums a reputation as an aberration in the history of mental health care, an arena for reckless physicians to experiment with invasive and dangerous treatments without inconveniences such as patient consent or clinical accountability. But not all asylums deserved this reputation. As early as 1796, William Tuke, a Quaker businessman, had founded a religious community asylum in York that rejected all physicality, whether as a means of restraint or of therapy.

The 'moral treatment' method pioneered by Tuke offered a gentler, alternative regime. It was not immediately heralded as a eureka moment, but the moral method grew quietly in repute, steadily spreading to become a template model from which many asylums elsewhere took their example in the nineteenth and twentieth centuries.

Daily routines in the moral treatment asylums were predicated on worship and work, replicating the characteristics of the wholesome, god-fearing lifestyle idealised in Tuke's time. Work may have been in the kitchens, the laundry, or the gardens but all patients would have made some contribution to the community. Mealtimes and worship created fixed points around which the staff hoped an orderly, healthy and sociable existence could be maintained. Restraint was replaced with vigilance and coercion with compassion, in the belief that a disciplined but humane regime offered better hopes for recovery than dehumanising alternatives. If order was preserved for long enough surely it would eventually become second nature; dormant moral faculties would be reactivated, and the capacity for independent self-discipline rekindled. Tuke believed that the potential for reason remained within even the most maddened of patients, and that punitive violence was counter-productive in the effort to reawaken it. As well as routine physical exercise, some moral asylums experimented with the creative therapies. Time was reserved each day for patients to write, sketch and paint – activities considered beneficial to mental health as potential outlets for emotion. In 1845 the institution in law of the 'Lunacy Commission' reinforced this progress by creating an inspectorate charged with stamping out the worst asylum abuses, further compelling disreputable institutions to clean up their act. Across the Channel, too, reforms instigated by Philippe Pinel had been pulling in the same moral direction, earning Pinel his reputation as 'the man who unchained the insane' – something that he, assisted by Jean-Baptiste Pussin, did literally for patients under his charge at Bicêtre Hospital in 1793, when he ordered their iron shackles removed. Admiration for the moral stand and humane approach exhibited by Tuke and Pinel grew steadily, contributing to an iterative process that saw asylums operating more ethically as the nineteenth century progressed.

Aside from the moral debate about whether asylums should be gentle or coercive in character, in Britain it was clear by the turn of the twentieth century that the original policy objective set for them – shifting mental ill health out of communities and into institutions – had been achieved. On the most superficial measure of sheer numbers of people incarcerated it had been achieved emphatically; in the century after the Criminal Lunatics Act had been passed in 1800 the institutionalised population of England had risen tenfold from about 10,000 to 100,000.[5] This rapid increase mirrored trends throughout Europe and America, impacting millions worldwide over the period.

As in England following James Hadfield's attempted assassination of George III, criminal case law influenced the course of developments in the United States. After two decades of living uneasily with the trauma haunting him in the aftermath of the American Civil War, James Garfield was shot in 1881 by Charles Guiteau, becoming the second serving US President to be assassinated. The subsequent trial did not edify the nascent discipline of psychiatry. Guiteau's guilt was not in doubt, but psychiatrists appearing in his defence argued for leniency on the grounds of mental ill health, describing their client as a disturbed 'degenerate', and the fallout ratcheted up populist clamour for yet greater incarceration of the mentally ill in the interests of public safety. Guiteau's case was also co-opted to provide ammunition for those going so far as to petition for the forced sterilisation of the mentally ill, an idea that sidestepped natural revulsion to become a serious medical proposition in America well before the Nazis adopted it as policy. But by far the biggest impact of Guiteau's trial was to galvanise afresh the pace of American institutionalisation, precipitating a deluge that surpassed even the European example. French historian and philosopher Michel Foucault suggested that the 'Great Confinement' of nineteenth-century Western institutionalisation, massive and supranational as it was, amounted to a calculated strategy to segregate the inconvenient, the eccentric and the idle poor away from society – a thinly veiled policy of deliberate social engineering.

In the history of madness, two events signal this change with singular clarity: in 1657, the founding of the Hôpital Général, and the Great Confinement of the poor; and in 1794, the liberation of the mad in chains at Bicêtre. Between these two singular and symmetrical events, something happened, whose ambiguity has perplexed historians of medicine: blind repression in an absolutist regime.[6]

Accepting mass institutionalisation as an internationally concerted, Machiavellian connivance feels a stretch. But even if social engineering was not the conscious objective, many among the huge numbers sequestered away were poorer people for whom institutionalisation was not necessary purely on the grounds of their mental health. They were human collateral of mission creep, caught in the net, committed and forgotten, as asylums swelled beyond their original remit of treating the mentally ill, to assume also the mantle of default domiciles for troublesome people who may or may not have been psychologically unwell but had issues with criminality or vice. New victims of old difficulties with knowing where an invisible line should be drawn.

Although there is much to decry in the record of mass institutionalisation, the movement did bring an accidental silver lining. The vast network of asylums built to relocate the mentally ill away from communities became hot house environments, helping to nurture medical understanding. The abundance of sufferers concentrated in asylums offered unprecedented opportunities for comparative observations in close quarters and at scale, aiding the process of grouping narrowly distinct sets of symptoms, and so greasing the wheels of classification and diagnosis. Such opportunities would not have been so readily available had the afflicted remained dispersed. As public disapprobation increasingly condemned the more egregious methods of restraint and control practised in asylums an imperative was also created to find better, more effective treatments. Asylums provided pioneer psychoanalysts and psychotherapists with a literal captive audience to help find those treatments, and in this environment necessity once again proved the mother of invention, albeit invention built on heaps of human misery. In this perverse way the asylums offered the full set of means, motive and opportunity to ease the passage towards the birth of psychiatry. Indeed, the Association of Medical Officers for Asylums and Hospitals for the Insane was formed in England in 1841, before later rebranding as the Royal Medico-Psychological Association and eventually, in 1971, becoming the Royal College of Psychiatrists; in the United States, meanwhile, the Association for Medical Superintendents of American Institutions for the Insane, established in 1844, was the direct forerunner of today's American Psychiatric Association.

Deinstitutionalisation

From the mid-twentieth century a slew of developments began to reverse the tide of a hundred years earlier by ushering an exodus away from the asylums and back into communities. Groundswell support for deinstitutionalisation was amplified by a deluge of disturbing personal testimonies from former internees, people like Urban Metcalf who offered up horrifying descriptions of their experiences in asylums. Some alleged that their incarceration had not been justified in the first place, insisting that their supposed mental struggles were mere fabrications conceived by ill-disposed family or business adversaries who simply desired their removal. Compounding the long-standing allegations of unethical practices, this spectre of indiscriminate, de facto imprisonment – or asylums as a method of circumventing trial by jury for those able to manipulate the system – stirred serious disquiet.

Weighing the accuracy of these many grievances we run into the perennial counter-argument – what else would you expect the mad and the paranoid to say? At a century or two's distance it would take a brave person to nail colours to a mast and proclaim judgement in any individual case. But by the mid-twentieth century discomforting allegations were piling up at a pace that could no longer be ignored, each one chipping away at public confidence in institutionalisation and lending momentum to the search for alternatives. In parallel, complementary work in academic and therapeutic understanding was pulling in the same direction. As Freudian ideas grew in popularity, old definitions of 'madness' were overhauled. Acceptance that occasional symptoms of mental ill health can fall within the natural psychological variations of many ordinary people spread through the Western world. For this great mass of low-level cases the model of indefinite detention in an asylum was shown up clearly as being like a hammer to a nut. As the metaphorical walls that had hitherto separated the 'mad' as 'the other' were being pulled down, inevitably the real world walls of bricks and mortar that physically closeted so many away in asylums would have to follow. As George Bernard Shaw wryly observed, 'An asylum for the sane would be empty in America.'[7]

In 1948 the single biggest revolution in the history of British healthcare provision arrived with the incorporation of the National Health Service. Before the advent of the NHS, death in childbirth, infant mortality and poor sanitation remained major problems bedevilling the nation, with healthcare a luxury available only to those who could pay. The post-war spirit demanded change, and Nye Bevan's legislation delivered it, creating a national health system founded on the principle of universal coverage and free at the point of access. Upon inception the NHS became immediately responsible for about a hundred asylums,[8] and was confronted with another pressing incentive for systemic change. By this time many of the Victorian and Edwardian mental health hospitals were a century old, crumbling into disrepair, and increasingly expensive to maintain. The search was on for a new, less financially burdensome option for accommodating their patients.

By 1954 Winston Churchill's Conservative government had established the Percy Commission, tasked with reviewing the legislative framework governing care and accommodation of the mentally ill. Three years later a central pillar of its report was a recommendation that psychiatric hospitals should be run with as much fidelity as possible to the model of 'normal' hospitals. This included an expectation that patients should not stay with them indefinitely, but rather should be working towards discharge and community resettlement. No longer would commitment to a mental institution be a one-way ticket. The Percy Report was one of a series of events that collectively eased back the frontiers of institutionalisation in the post-war years. The 1959 Mental Health Act removed promiscuity as legal grounds for incarceration, and it is incredible to reflect that it was considered sufficient justification right up to the cusp of 1960s sexual liberation. Then, in 1961, speaking to the National Association for Mental Health, Enoch Powell outlined the government's plans to introduce a community-based model of care for mental health patients to replace the old dependence on asylums. Ambitions were set out to reduce the number of psychiatric beds by 75,000, and close most institutions within fifteen years.

> We have to strive to alter our whole mentality about hospitals and about mental hospitals especially. Hospital building is not like pyramid building, the erection of memorials to endure to a remote posterity. We have to get the idea into our heads that a hospital is a shell, a framework, however complex, to contain certain processes, and when the processes change or are superseded, then the shell must most probably be scrapped.[9]

This Conservative policy of scything back Britain's engorged asylum system survived into the Thatcher era, finding natural synergy with her administration's instinctive distaste for an unwieldy, interventionist welfare state. Across the Atlantic events once more unfolded in a similar vein to Britain, but in the United States deinstitutionalisation was more controversial, with some politicians seeking to connect the policy with the weeping sore that was the national debate over gun laws. President Trump responded to a question about gun control at a rally in New Hampshire in August 2019, caressing the issue with the delicate touch for which he is renowned:

> These people are mentally ill, and nobody talks about that …
> I think we have to start building institutions again because,

if you look at the '60s and '70s so many of these institutions were closed, and the people were just allowed to go on the streets.[10]

Trump may have been conflating criminality with mental illness, but he wasn't kidding about the American proclivity for institutions. At the statistical peak, some half a million people were incarcerated in American mental institutions in the 1950s[11] before a mass closure of mental hospitals in the second half of the twentieth century left fewer than 40,000 state psychiatric beds by the turn of the millennium,[12] the vestigial remnants of an apparently bygone age. But when the asylums closed their doors in the United States, spilling vast numbers of formerly incarcerated mentally ill people back into communities, they did so into a very different systemic context from the United Kingdom, where community services waited to plug at least some of the gaps. The capacity of the National Health Service remains far from ideal, but it at least offers a safety net, irrespective of ability to pay. In the US, with the asylums gone and a layered, insurance-based system of Medicare and Medicaid coverage that remains well short of universal, affordable access to mental health care is beyond the reach of many Americans. The United States has a particular challenge managing people with psychological issues who are unable to get the help they need and, in their desperate isolation, may present a risk to themselves and others.

The Psychopharmacological Revolution

On both sides of the Atlantic, mass transition away from asylums and into communities was eased along by the psychopharmacological revolution. A plethora of new drugs, developed in the 1950s and 1960s, helped control the moods of unstable patients, lessening the need for monumental institutions to do the job instead. At a time when talking therapies remained embryonic, these developmental drugs offered the only pragmatic alternative to asylums, and the wave of mass deinstitutionalisation was borne along on chemical tides. The first psychotropic drugs appeared in the early 1950s and were initially targeted at manic depression. From there, the range and scope of available drugs quickly ballooned and by the 1970s Valium, otherwise known as diazepam, had become established as the world's most frequently prescribed medication bar none.[13] Provided that dosages were maintained these drugs made it possible for people to leave the confines of mental health hospitals to resume their places in society, where they could be managed on an outpatient basis, bringing immense savings to the state. While prescribing drugs in huge quantities carries a financial cost, it remains far cheaper than building, staffing and maintaining a vast institutional infrastructure.

The psychopharmacological revolution is one of the most important advances in the history of mental health care, bringing containment and comfort to many, but it has not been free of controversy. There is a question of scale. A 2019 publication from Public Health England reported that there are some 7.3 million people regularly taking anti-depressants in England alone.[14] 930,000 have been taking them consistently for more than three years,[15] and so these people's relationship with the drugs extends beyond a temporary crutch; they have received them into their established routines. This trend of anti-depressant drug consumption becoming normalised within everyday life is even more pronounced in America, where 25 million adults have been on the drugs for at least two years and 15 million for more than five years, a rate that has tripled since the millennium according to a 2018 Analysis of Federal Data conducted by the *New York Times*.[16] These statistics not only exceed but dwarf by orders of magnitude the numbers ever held in asylums in either country, demonstrating how the reach of prescription medication has proved more penetrative than the tendrils of the old asylum system – a system which also, by its nature, existed on the edge of society, an orbiting appendage that may have impacted thousands but never became an intrinsic feature of the day-to-day life for millions in all walks of life.

The Western predilection for medication shows no signs of waning, and the range of psychological ailments catered for by pharmacology has expanded markedly, now encompassing mild to moderate mental ill health issues alongside the more severe conditions that were its original focus. Pills are now a familiar, albeit sometimes unspoken, part of the day-to-day routine for millions. But when repeat prescriptions rack up year on year, in a pattern that extends over several years and perhaps even a patient's whole lifetime, inevitable questions about addiction and oversubscription arise. Can indefinite dependence really be the best path? Or is it just the path of least resistance, an expedient for busy GPs and an easy choice for all of us? The option to manage symptoms through medication, to the point where people can 'get by', can reinforce the understandable reluctance of some patients to confront issues directly, perhaps via therapy, even though the latter may be the better long-term option. Although talking therapies and medication are not perfect substitutes in the economic sense, the scale of medication has given rise to a healthy debate about the respective places of prescription drugs and talking therapies in an optimally configured response to mental ill health. Medicating people is not just cheaper than maintaining an asylum, it is cheaper than talking therapies too. Putting a therapist through the years of training needed for them to practise, then bearing the costs of their salaries, supervision and continuing professional development is a major commitment for any state to contemplate. Publicly organised talking therapy services also attract considerable overheads, way before a patient arrives in a room and in front of a therapist. In the absence of adequately funded therapy services people needing talking therapies may face a long wait, and in this context medics making assessment and triage decisions, selecting from the toolkit available, may naturally show a high propensity to turn to prescription medication as the default choice. If the only tool you can access is a hammer, it is tempting to treat everything as if it were a nail. But indefinite medication is not a perfect solution that best meets all mental health needs. Nevertheless, it should be acknowledged that pharmacological advances have contributed much to the long battle for mental health, providing a weapon that, in the twenty-first century, is sparing many who might have been condemned to asylums in times past.

Anti-psychiatry

In the sea-change decades that followed the war, as treatment orthodoxies were morphing and the exodus from asylums gathered pace, a sceptical 'anti-psychiatry' movement was also on the rise. The anti-psychiatrists found many grievances with conventional psychotherapy. Adherents held that the power imbalance between doctors and patients had created a system little better than a coercive instrument of oppression marred by subjective diagnosis and ineffective treatments. Credence for such thinking was gifted added momentum by the abuses of the asylum era and the notorious treatments associated with it. But the anti-psychiatrists went further than merely criticising clear errors and abuses by questioning the very status of psychiatry as a legitimate medical specialism. Hard won though that status had been, the anti-psychiatrists thought it ill deserved, arguing that psychiatry was a damaging sham propagated by an establishment of charlatans guilty of medicalising what was, in actuality, just normal human behaviour. They reserved special criticism for what they considered injudiciously reckless proliferation of psychiatric drugs, particularly in cases where prescriptions were made out to young children.

The term 'anti-psychiatry' was first used by David Cooper in 1967, and fellow psychiatrists R. D. Laing, Thomas Szasz, Theodore Lidz and Silvano Arieti became prominent disciples of the movement. Collectively they revived old criticisms about the subjective difficulty of where to draw the line that divides normal and abnormal behaviour, claiming that the symptoms medics would leap on as being indicative of schizophrenia and psychosis were, in fact, normal facets of the human response when trying to cope with extreme circumstances in imperfect societies – 'a rational adjustment [to] an insane world',[17] as Laing himself has been quoted as putting it. He believed that 'the experience and behaviour that gets labelled as schizophrenia is a special strategy that the patient invents in order to live with an unliveable situation'[18].

Psychosis, it was alleged, was a defence mechanism – part of a healing process, and as such something that medics should not seek to inhibit. Instead sufferers ought to be encouraged to explore their true nature to the fullest expression, living out manic episodes to their extremes in order to achieve the best prospects for recovery. Madness, as Laing also said, 'need not be all breakdown; it may also be break-through'.[19] When it came to theories of causation, Laing argued vigorously that it was society – and especially the schizophrenic patient's immediate family – that was responsible for the deviant behaviour they exhibited, which was then erroneously labelled as mental illness and only worsened by subsequent treatment within the flawed institution system. Laing considered poor parenting to be a major risk factor for schizophrenia in particular. Foucault, the vehement critic of institutionalisation, found kindred spirits in the ranks of anti-psychiatrists. He argued that psychiatry, like the asylums, was primarily a tool of social control. Mass confinement and the chains of physical restraint had long been the preferred methods for asserting that control, before being replaced by drugs and speciously therapeutic mechanisms for internalising that oppression in the later twentieth century. But though the methods had changed, in his view the object of psychiatry remained the same: control. In his 1961 work *Madness and Civilization: A History of Insanity in the Age of Reason*, Foucault critiques the medical framework and the established corpus of received psychological wisdom as no more than a moveable feast of insanity, liable to bend with the wind according to the social mores of the age.

After enjoying an initial flash of popularity, many of the anti-psychiatry movement's ideas proved unpalatable with the passage of time, and its adherents were relegated to the professional fringe. The movement's reputation was further tarnished by its popularity with Scientologists, who co-opted some of its ideas within their own philosophy. In later life even Laing himself eventually became disillusioned with his former views, remarking to an interviewer, 'I was looked to as one who had the answers, but I never had them.'[20] For the loved ones of people suffering from schizophrenia, the anti-psychiatrist theory of familial culpability must have been particularly distressing. It was a suggestion that risked families being stigmatised, and risked sufferers being removed from loving, home environments into less supportive, potentially more dangerous circumstances. The eagerness of the anti-psychiatry movement to dismiss psychosis and schizophrenia as normal also risked any associated disruptive behaviour being interpreted as criminal rather than medical, and so the province of the justice system rather than medicine. Despite these unintended, regressive consequences it is notable that most advocates of anti-psychiatry, even those who questioned the very reality of mental illness, remained supportive of talking therapies. In a perverse way the movement also engendered greater acceptance that many mental health issues are rooted in a combination of biological, psychological and social components, or 'biopsychosocial factors' in today's industry terminology – a holistic perspective that has been of great benefit to achieving a more holistic understanding of human health.

7

INDUSTRY AND INSIGHT –
MENTAL HEALTH AND GLOBALISED
CAPITALISM

Industrial Revolution & Social Upheaval

'Man is born free and everywhere he is in chains.'[1] These opening lines of Jean-Jacques Rousseau's *Social Contract* were first published in 1762, on the threshold of an Industrial Revolution in England and a political revolution, more bloodied in nature, in France. It challenged the divine right of hereditary monarchs to absolute rule, arguing instead for the rights of individuals to determine the laws by which they are governed, within a system of basic democratic and economic equality, freedoms and protections. As the ideas raised by the *Social Contract* were finding sympathy throughout Europe, the Industrial Revolution, spanning roughly 1760 to 1840, was also getting into stride. It fired the starting pistol on a chain of events that reshaped the world. From its origins in water and steam and a transition from manual processes to rudimentary mechanisation in the textile mills of Britain, the Industrial Revolution ushered in a sequence of advancements in rail, road, commerce and trade that saw business routinely transacted across international boundaries and on ever greater scales. Once the industrial genie was out of the bottle, it radiated into ever more complex supply and distribution chains, seminal developments in electronics and aviation, the diversification of financial commodities, the rise and fall of Wall Street, and gaining in spite of all setbacks the breathless pace that propelled humanity onwards into a modern world of globalised, interconnected trade, with a ferocious momentum that can only really be conveyed in an excessively lengthy, inadequately punctuated sentence.

As these forces grew massive in scale, nations shook with accompanying political and social upheaval. The question of how societies should be organised to generate and distribute the wealth created by the changes afoot was sharply pressing. In the *Social Contract*, Rousseau sketched out his conception of the 'general will', an inclusive vision for direct democracy with a franchise incorporating men and women alike. The social contract, he argued, should be a covenant establishing the relationship between society and the individual, within a system that protected everyone equally under the law. These progressive ideas were radical for the time but were not exclusive to Rousseau or France. Thomas Hobbes' *Leviathan*, the 1651 antecedent of Rousseau's work, deliberated the same issues of statecraft.

He described three options for organising the state, or 'commonwealth': monarchy, aristocracy and democracy. Hobbes favoured monarchy on the grounds that it offered fewer opportunities for corruption and decay. But Hobbes' deliberations reflected the fact that other possibilities were once again occupying serious minds in the seventeenth century, perhaps for the first time in centuries in European nations where monarchy had seemed the only conceivable form of government since Roman times. Indeed, *Leviathan* was published very shortly after tensions had erupted into England's Civil War, fought over the balance of authority between Parliament and the Crown, which only ended when Charles I was separated from his head in 1649, ushering in the interregnum period when England, Scotland and Ireland briefly became a republic.

Across the Channel the French also saw social unrest ascend to a bloody crescendo when their revolution arrived in 1789, within decades of Rousseau's own warnings. The French Revolution brought into terrible relief the very real risks of poverty, inequality and civil rights frustrated combusting amid the growing pains of industrialising societies. In France, the intensely turbulent period from 1789 to 1794 witnessed the execution of a king, the disestablishment of the Catholic Church and the rise of Robespierre and the Reign of Terror, as the guillotine was liberally employed in an aggressive roll-out of the revolutionary ideals of *liberté, égalité and fraternité*. But as the Revolution ended, supplies of these ideals appeared to have been exhausted gaining the victory, and France too lurched from monarchy to republic, then quickly to dictatorship under the leadership of Napoleon Bonaparte, with huge consequences for all of Europe. The revolutionary terror unleashed was felt in the breast of ruling elites right across the continent. A century and a half on from the monarchy's restoration, England was again a tinderbox close by the time of the 1819 massacre at Peterloo, where popular demands for parliamentary reform were met with a cavalry charge.

In its wake, the events in France were perceived more and more as a bloody example of the risks run when the 'social contract' was not honoured, when poverty and injustice went unchecked. If revolution could happen there, why not elsewhere? Why not in England a second time? Could any of Europe's crowned heads feel safe? In the light of these fears, Rousseau's ideological questions about freedoms and the balance of power assumed ever higher consequence. A new settlement was needed. In the following century, as nations sought different angles to grasp these issues, flirtations with communism and fascism were ushered in with polemic of equal vigour by advocates on either side. Russia succumbed to its own revolution in 1917, replacing the Romanovs with decades of Bolshevism, Stalinism and Soviet communism, while further west the malign ingredients that would one day permit a new, National Socialist ideology to gain a foothold in a unified Germany were also falling into place.

All the while the wheels of early industrialisation continued to accelerate. Into this new world of international commerce a new and powerful player emerged: the multinational corporation. In time, big business would accrue power to rival monarchs and even nation states

in influence, a new player to disrupt and complicate the political and social balance of power. Thomas Hobbes might have seen his way clear to acknowledging a fourth agent of social control had he been writing two centuries later. These new multinationals enriched many, but their wealth could also make them dangerous when permitted to operate unfettered by regulation, something their unprecedented international reach made difficult. Their sheer size also meant that problems, when they came, created tremors on a scale hitherto unseen. An early example had arrived in the 1770s when the East India Company, one of the first super-powered corporations, which at its peak oversaw more than a third of Britain's trade,[2] took down thirty invested banks across Europe upon its collapse. The East India Company was the world's first multinational, giving a taste of things to come in the globalist age of powerful corporate behemoths and bringing systemic risks described by William Dalrymple in *The Anarchy*:

> The East India Company remains today history's most ominous warning about the potential abuse of corporate power and the insidious means by which the interests of shareholders can seemingly become those of the state. When worries are voiced today about the power of corporations and the way global companies can find ways around the laws and the legislatures of individual nation states, it is no accident that they sound like eighteenth-century commentators such as Horace Walpole, who decried the way East India Company wealth had corrupted parliament.[3]

For every organisation that rose high, faltered and fell, the invisible hand[4] of the free market, animated by the profit incentive and equipped with the rapidly expanding toolkit of industrialisation, created another to take its place. Networks of commerce grew and grew, and when the world wars of 1914 to 1918 and 1939 to 1945 disrupted this trajectory, the flames of human progress dimmed but were not extinguished. The necessities of wartime even accelerated development in some spheres, adding impetus to the rate of technological progress, and once humanity's appetite for military applications of 'the lights of perverted science',[5] as Churchill described them, had passed, the peacetime potential of new technologies was ripe to be unleashed. But the disruptions of war had corroded, or wiped away altogether, many old-world structures of social, political and economic organisation, creating a fresh canvas on which new designs could be painted.

After the Second World War

So how would nation states be organised in the new world? Under what political and economic model would new scientific and technological genius, and the powerhouse multinationals thriving on it, best be marshalled? Would the social contract be respected? As the war drew to a close the 'big three' of Stalin, Roosevelt and Churchill met in conference at Yalta and at Potsdam to plan its denouement, carving out an agreement for the post-war world order. With the collapse of the Third Reich fascism was discredited, the chiefs who had nurtured it dead and disgraced. The Iron Curtain soon descended, with the Berlin

Wall, erected by the Soviets in 1961, putting communism on the other side of the looking glass from the capitalist West. The aftermath of the war also gave rise to the United Nations, established in 1945 as a bulwark intended to prevent a recurrence of the devastation of the recent past. Into this environment, and nourished by the Marshall Plan, the exhausted and impoverished Western nations set about the task of rebuilding their battle-scarred physical landscapes, societies and economies in the post-war decades. Like the seed that survives the frozen months below ground, the busy networks of global trade and interconnectedness that had come into being before the wars, only to be forced into retreat by the catastrophes that followed, re-emerged and resumed course towards full expression.

Neoliberal Democracy

Having rejected the totalitarian extremes of fascism and communism, the main political parties of the West bunched into a narrow space, easing into a new hegemony of liberal democracy, coupled with 'neoliberal' economics, that would come to dominate Western societies. These democracies shared features designed to offer protection against the resurgence of political extremism, a priority of the Yalta delegates as they manoeuvred to secure lasting peace. Universal suffrage, a vibrant civil sphere and freedom of the press and religion became the building blocks of Western societies, all predicated on a neoliberal economic model characterised by free trade and the rejection of overblown state interference – conditions that succeeded in incubating free corporate interests to a degree that would have been unconscionable east of the Berlin Wall. In the post-war decades, Western political debate was reduced to squabbles at the margins over a few percentage points of difference in manipulation of tax, spend, interest rates and the more minor economic levers. Even within this narrow band, legislators in the late twentieth and early twenty-first century increasingly inclined towards deregulation, hoping to promote growth by creating conditions where markets were free to operate in a context of reasonable – but not stultifying – taxation. In so doing successive generations of politicians were seeking the Goldilocks zone where enterprise and profits, taxation and public investment are harmoniously optimised, with the aim of creating economies that steadily generated demand, and so jobs, and so more demand – facilitating a virtuous 'trickle down' of wealth, and a socially acceptable balance between the rewards accruing from enterprise and the tax receipts accruing to governments and so available for redistribution. In this way, it was hoped, prosperity and social cohesion could both be sustained.

This neoliberal economic model found particular political enthusiasm in the time of Thatcher and Reagan, as the 1980s witnessed the waxing power of big business. By then neoliberal thinking had become so entrenched in the West that when the last viable alternative faltered, as the seams holding together the Soviet states began to fray near the decade's end, the ideological debate over how best to organise human affairs appeared to have been conclusively settled. For communism, the red flags were everywhere, and by 1989 American political scientist Francis Fukuyama was ready to announce that the fall of the Berlin Wall and collapse of the Soviet Union presaged 'not just the end of the cold war, or the passing of a particular period of post-war history, but the end of history as such: That is, the end-point of mankind's ideological evolution and the universalization of Western liberal democracy as the final form of human government'.[6]

With communism's bolt apparently shot, the world was indeed seemingly converging on the neoliberal model with irresistible momentum. Even when parties traditionally associated with heavier programmes of tax-and-spend subsequently returned to power, the price of achieving it was policy that sacrificed their leftist heritage in favour of the new centre ground. When Labour swept into office after the 1997 election it was Blair's New Labour philosophy that won the party its mandate to govern, with a manifesto so long on business-friendly rhetoric as to bring howls from a Keir Hardie or Ramsay MacDonald had they been around to see it. Any ardent socialist or extreme right-winger of the earlier twentieth century, granted a window through time, might have gazed upon the modern political debate and declared de facto consensus – barely an inch of daylight separating the parties' trajectories as they all eyed the same narrow landing zone. For better or worse, the course was fixed; the conditions that would nurture the generations reaching adulthood in the twenty-first century had been established.

Globalisation and Mental Health

The link between our economic circumstances and our health outcomes is now well established,[7] so understanding today's economic dynamics and how they came to be is necessary if we are to comprehend the suggested modern epidemic – and where it might go next. In terms of mental health, the big questions now are 'What have been the impacts of industrialisation, capitalism, and globalisation on our psychological health?' and 'Is the dominant, neoliberal political and economic model that defines the societies we now live in well suited to well-being?'

When the storm of the Second World War cleared, the first shoots of very different-looking European labour markets emerged from the ashes. In the UK, as the need to supply the Allied war machine vanished abruptly, the labour market shifted away from manufacturing and towards a more office-oriented model. A desk-driven economy, powered by legions of workers dedicating forty hours a week to their computers, is a new phenomenon in evolutionary terms. The main stage of human endeavour shifted from the agricultural, to the industrial, to the office over a period spanning just a handful of generations. If the agricultural and industrial arenas had shared one common characteristic, it was sweat. The growth of the service industries, and the rise of computing on an accelerating curve, changed all this in the Western economies. For millions of hunter-gatherer *Homo sapiens*, a daily commute to the office followed by several hours of physical inactivity became the new routine; sedentary a newly normalised lifestyle option. It is an option that was not so readily available to preceding generations, living when work largely meant physical labour, or even further back when the need to hurry after food, or away from woolly predators, demanded at least some exertion from their ancestors' animalistic biology. Could this new lifestyle have exercised an enervating effect on millions, spreading an ennui that could not have proliferated when employment remained weighted towards the physical trades? Has the technological evolution's fevered pace outstripped our capacity to adapt? There *is* a physical aspect to human emotions: exercise stimulates production and release of mood-lifting endorphins in the brain's hypothalamus and pituitary gland, and a host of studies have shown the link between exercise and positive mood.[8] Our naturally active, agile human bodies are the product of thousands of years adjusting to the demands of our environment, and any biological organism suddenly displaced into an unfamiliar environment will require time to adapt. Perhaps the hypothesised modern epidemic of mental ill health is simply what happens when the active patterns of the world we knew are swept away, and hastily replaced with a static *modus vivendi* so alien to our constitutions that nature could not have anticipated it.

Following humanity's migration to the office, the latter part of the twentieth century witnessed ever greater geographical dispersion of supply and distribution chains, and ever bigger cash values of imports and exports. The world shrank while big business, incubated in the post-war neoliberal hegemony, grew. With money and power inexorably gravitating towards large corporations, inequality has become increasingly stretched. Availability of cheap labour from all over the world, along with the increased bargaining power of huge multinationals, has acted to suppress wage growth for most workers in Western economies. China has turned outwards to become a more active participant in international trade. When a nation boasting a quarter of the world's population ceases to be a sleeping giant and awakens to flex its muscles, rising to compete with the established economies, the process will release major shock waves into those economies. And it was not just China; in the latter part of the twentieth century a raft of tiger economies surged through the gears on their own journeys up the international pecking order, ramping up competition and disrupting the economic hierarchy. In the United Kingdom and the United States, existential threats from new competition and new technology alike rendered traditionally powerful industries no longer viable – major sectors like mining, shipbuilding and steel. As the consequent flight from industry and rebalancing of labour markets began to bite, governments faced the dilemma of whether to intervene with tariffs and subsidies to protect sickly domestic industries that were becoming uncompetitive on their own terms. But under the laissez-faire neoliberal doctrine, inefficient enterprises must be allowed to fail if they cannot stand the glare of competition. As new comparative advantages emerge, the old are cast adrift and lost. Like a living organism shedding dead skin, this is considered a good thing in the long term. But while this argument may stack up in abstract in a classroom, for a generation in the northern industrial heartlands of Britain and the Rust Belt of America it did nothing to lessen the pain of living through the process as their leaders left the market to take its course. The resulting impoverishment has yet to be overcome in some communities, and if the strategic case for modernisation was undeniable, so too was the case to have better mitigated the human collateral.

As global capitalism has reached maturity, with the world's economies now connected like a giant nervous system, there is more scope for disturbance in one part of the complex network to undermine the rest – particularly when that disturbance strikes a major keystone. As the saying goes, when America sneezes, the world catches cold.⁹ In the new millennium, the heavily interlinked economies of the West would discover what happens when international tectonic forces more powerful than ever legislated for erupt into a vulnerable, nationally oriented competitive system ill equipped to handle them. With enough pressure, plates eventually shift and there is always an earthquake. In 2007, the banking crisis hit. The first phase of what many economists would later judge the worst financial crash since the 1930s had ground into motion, and terms like 'Sub-Prime', 'Over Leveraged', and 'Bank Run' became staples of news bulletins the world over, quickly followed by 'Quantitative Easing', 'Bail Out' and 'Austerity' as the Old Lady of Threadneedle Street, the Federal Reserve and legislators scrambled to respond. When these convulsions subsided, a period of low growth descended on the Western economies and would remain for a decade. Since the financial crisis, this weak growth has gone hand in hand with stagnant wage rates. Unlike the experience of previous generations, when one wage was often enough to support a whole family, many households today find themselves requiring multiple income streams just to stand still.

In the fallout of the financial crisis a new fashion for a creative mode of engaging employees emerged – or perhaps not quite employees, as the line is a bit grey on 'zero-hours contracts'. According to data from the UK Office of National Statistics, the number of people on zero-hours contracts rose from 150,000 at the onset of the economic shock in 2008 to some 896,000 by 2019.[10] Flexible working may suit some, but for people taking short-term berths out of necessity, how is your tolerance for uncertainty? It can easily be imagined that living hand to mouth and paycheque to paycheque might involve more anxiety than the 'job for life', when finding one remained a realistic prospect.

Following the banking crisis, those banks that survived reacted to having been exposed as hopelessly overleveraged at its onset by recoiling too far in the other direction. Lending criteria tightened to an absurd degree. In combination with suppressed wage rates and rise of the 'gig' economy, this pushed the dream of home ownership out of reach for many. In 1979 the average house price in England and Wales was three times the average wage. By 2019 the multiple had risen to more than seven times,[11] a market failure crying out for intervention that is still awaited. The nervousness of banks to serve their normal lending function after the crash also paved the way for the short-lived heyday of the payday loans companies. People who found themselves unable to access credit through traditional routes were pushed into the arms of these cowboy lenders, with punishing interest rates and collection methods. They precipitated a flood of despairing victims into mental health services before their Wild West freedoms were eventually curbed by legislation. In this climate of rising personal debt, combined with a shortage of affordable housing, homelessness has become increasingly problematic. Rough sleeping is on the rise.[12] Some say money can't buy happiness – but some should try being cheerful without even enough money to keep a roof over their heads. Life without a home is miserable, and lack of a fixed address brings a lack of stability that heightens a whole raft of secondary risks, poorer mental health included. Safe, permanent accommodation not only gives a security that is vital to peace of mind, but also acts as a gateway to social inclusion and basic services, making it easier to remain registered with a GP and so to gain an onward referral to other health services beyond that. Lack of a consistent home and other life structures not only makes mental ill health more likely, but also makes it harder for mental health professionals to help when things do go wrong, with no fixed foundations to build upon. Mental health issues increase the risk of homelessness, and homelessness increases the risk of enduring mental ill health.

Recessions happen, of course, but it is now clear that, since the banking crisis, neoliberal economics has been experiencing a particularly twenty-first-century-shaped wobble. This is the turbulent stage that has welcomed an ingénue generation of millennials into adulthood, young adults who have, through a combination of necessity and expedience, delayed key events such as home ownership, marriage and children, the major milestones that anchor life's journey. It is an economic context that has left many feeling hopeless. When getting on in life does not seem feasible, when upward social mobility is not realistic, people become frustrated – their wheels spinning, full of 'sound and fury' that is 'signifying nothing',[13] because nothing is possible. This predicament has left life feeling unpleasantly rudderless for many among 'Generation Rent', and the turbulence only looks like getting worse now that economies are also being forced to grapple with the financial fallout of the Covid-19 pandemic.

So what is the verdict on the contribution of modern liberal democracy and twenty-first-century, Western-style capitalism to the happiness bottom line? Has neoliberalism breached the parameters of Rousseau's social contract? It has ushered the market into every aspect of twenty-first-century life; consumerism is more powerful than ever in the modern attention economy. But the idea of society as a universal market, rather than the old Greek conception of a *polis* or civil community of interests, is one that demands careful navigation. If we think of people too much as counted consumption and production beans we may think too little of their inherent human value – a worth that cannot be measured in pounds and pence. The negative impacts of full-tilt free-market forces on the mental health of some has been amplified by its coinciding with the weakening of traditional counterbalances: the slow atrophy of faith and spiritual measures of human value, which kept the economic ones from being not only the primary but virtually the *only* currency by which society places value on anything. Capitalism has undoubtedly enriched us materially and in aggregate, but we must be careful how the process is shepherded along, mitigating the collateral damage on those left behind. The integrity of society is risked when the material enrichment neoliberalism has delivered is not felt sufficiently by everyone. American Nobel Prize-winning economist Joseph Stiglitz described the relationship between economics and wellness, offering a warning that the free-market profit incentive alone is no guarantee of maximising societal well-being, and outlining an alternative vision for corralling the benefits of modern market economies:

> The other vision is of a society where the gap between the haves and the have-nots has been narrowed, where there is a sense of shared destiny, a common commitment to opportunity and fairness, where the words 'liberty and justice for all' actually mean what they seem to mean, where we take seriously the Universal Declaration of Human Rights, which emphasizes the importance not just of civil rights but of economic rights, and not just the rights of property but the economic rights of ordinary citizens. In this vision, we have an increasingly vibrant political system far different from the one in which eighty percent of the young are so alienated that they don't even bother to vote. I believe that this second vision is the only one that is consistent with our heritage and our values. In it the well-being of our citizens—and even our economic growth, especially if properly measured—will be much higher than what we can achieve if our society remains deeply divided.[14]

In articulating this vision perhaps Stiglitz is only reminding us of a latent truth that we may now have forgotten, but that some once knew in a time before high-end capitalism, before industrialisation, and before even the long centuries of direct monarchical rule:

> Then none was for a party;
> Then all were for the state;
> Then the great man helped the poor,
> And the poor man loved the great;
> Then lands were fairly portioned;
> Then spoils were fairly sold;
> The Romans were like brothers, in the brave days of old[15]

The free market now stands accused of being impotent in the face of the big modern challenges, inequality and climate change uppermost among them. Globalisation has raised the biggest multinationals to the status of stateless superpowers, but trickle-down economics is in danger of drying up in a world where corporations can cherry-pick a nominal headquarters on the basis of tax efficiency. With in-work poverty increasingly problematic and income inequality worsening,[16] neoliberalism's rising tide now looks underpowered and unequal to serving its traditional function of raising all boats. A metaphor involving locks might be needed to properly represent collective fleet manoeuvres today.

Perhaps it was not by design, but Western societies *are* now perilously close to breaching the social contact that Rousseau sought to define. Having ceded so much authority to an almost religious faith in the free market, legislators now appear toothless when major existential shocks demand action. The supercharged consumerist workaholic culture of high-end capitalism feels like an out-of-control train, and must be a contender for the second ingredient in the recipe for any modern epidemic of mental ill health. As would be expected with a runaway train, it is now failing to stop at too many platforms. The long-standing, productive partnership of liberal democracy and liberal economics is itself put at risk by this if dissatisfaction with inequality, along with apparent political inability to address climate change, undermines faith in the free market. The consequences of that could be about the most damaging prospect of all for human well-being if it causes another kneejerk to the extremes, because any properly balanced assessment of neoliberalism and its contribution to our collective 'happiness yield' must surely rank it in credit. Climate concerns aside, the burning issues at hand – poverty, inequality, and the balance of power – are the old familiars from the times of Rousseau, Robespierre and even the Romans. Since those times, and in spite of all criticism, the liberal democratic political system and the free market have delivered more for human health and advancement than any extreme, interventionist or totalitarian alternative attempted in history. Of all political and economic models it has the best record for promoting human welfare, whether through freedom, rights or economic enrichment. Time and again, across the globe, the invisible hand of free market forces has proved the most reliable vehicle for raising people from poverty, and in Britain it was the liberal democratic system that crystallised both the National Health Service and the welfare state. Neoliberalism's modern face, and our twenty-first-century economic dynamics, may undervalue the humanity and human emotions we need to centre ourselves, and are probably not perfectly configured for fostering well-being, but if neoliberalism has lost its way we might do well to remember why the Yalta delegates were so keen to avoid a return to the political extremes, and be careful about throwing out the global world order without first seeing what would follow. It is recalibration that is now required, not another revolution.

Modern Psychological Therapies

It has not been only trade flowing across national borders at increasing pace since the Industrial Revolution, but ideas too. Through the twentieth century, medical knowledge benefitted from a rich spirit of international academic co-operation and from cross-fertilisation of ideas in increasingly open flow. The American Psychiatric Association's *Diagnostic and Statistical Manual of Mental Disorders* (DSM) was first published in 1952, quickly becoming a 'bible of mental health' for many clinician practitioners. It helped bring desperately needed common definition and international standardisation to psychological health care, and through successive updates its editions have anchored the field worldwide. With these reference points established, the latter twentieth century witnessed a vast expansion in the granular understanding of more and more distinct mental health conditions, with ever more refined appreciation of their particular characteristics. This in turn cranked the throttle on a parallel expansion in the arsenal of evidence-based psychotherapeutic techniques available to combat them. A constellation of new therapies burst into being, earned their stripes and grew in repute to become staples of the psychotherapist's toolkit – family therapy, cognitive therapy and behavioural therapy among them. The light that had begun illuminating the murky new discipline of psychotherapy in the Renaissance continued to grow in size and radiance, to the great benefit of millions of patients worldwide.

Mental Health in Popular Culture

The twentieth century also delivered a radical overhaul in communications technologies, with the advent of radio, television and mass media offering fresh methods for reaching large audiences to influence public attitudes on a whole range of topics including mental health. Pop culture caught fire. The association between artistic creativity, tortured vulnerability and psychopathology that had piqued the interest of Cesare Lombroso endured, but the modern version assumed a sinister fatality. The anguish of sufferers played out in the public eye to be picked over and mythicised. Janice Joplin and Jimi Hendrix were dead by overdose aged twenty-seven, Heath Ledger was gone at twenty-eight, and Sid Vicious at just twenty-one. Marilyn Monroe died by her own hand aged thirty-six, Sylvia Plath at thirty, and Kurt Cobain put a shotgun to his head aged twenty-four. James Dean's death, also aged twenty-four, came in an accidental collision at the wheel of his Porsche Spyder, but he is another tortured icon of the twentieth century whose legend soared on the back of an early death. After coming dangerously close to glamorising the image of a fast life and an early demise, popular culture turned a corner towards the end of the millennium, finally getting to grips with the insidious stigma that had done so much to damage the cause of mental health. The message that it is okay not to feel okay finally cut through. It was helped to the eyes and ears of billions by the rise of another revolutionary force, one poised to change the world once again. But this would be a revolution unlike any that had gone before, orders of magnitude beyond even the Industrial Revolution in pace and in reach. This time the changes coming would propel humanity into an entirely new dimension.

8

WORLDWIDE WORRIES? – MENTAL HEALTH IN THE DIGITAL AGE

In 1971 a seemingly unremarkable event occurred in the working day of Raymond Tomlinson, a computer technician in Cambridge, Massachusetts. It did not shake the foundations of civilisation; its importance barely registered at the time, even with the unassuming Tomlinson. His quiet breakthrough was greeted with none of the shock and awe that accompanied the sack of Rome, the revolution in France, or any of the other seminal events eulogised as turning points in history textbooks. Nevertheless, it was an achievement with colossal repercussions that must surely see it ranked alongside these epic moments once the passage of time permits true perspective to be gauged. Because it was in 1971 that Tomlinson first transmitted electronic mail from one device to another over ARPANET, the forerunner of the internet. This inaugural node-to-node e-mail also marked the first occasion when an '@' sign was used to identify an intended recipient. In that moment, a Rubicon was crossed, and a digital revolution unleashed.

From these humble beginnings, developments in the domain of networks, nodes and nerds hastened on through the 1970s and 1980s, before the recognisable shape of our modern, digital world coalesced from the 'white heat of technological revolution',[1] as Harold Wilson had called it, towards the century's end. Personal computer ownership became increasingly affordable, quickly penetrating most households, and by the new millennium most of these devices were networked. By 2004 people using these networks were able to connect with friends on Facebook, and in 2005 they could even indulge these friends with videos of cats, after YouTube's own entry onto the digital stage. Even with a coup of that magnitude safely in the bag, digital innovation roared ever onwards, spawning new apps and new strains of social media on the way to becoming the ubiquitous feature of daily life it is today.

In parallel, technology was advancing hard on another front: telephony. Although mobile telephone communications had been around for decades, the first mass-produced handheld devices did not arrive until the 1970s. Even then, the old-style common or garden variety of static 'finger in the dial' rotary telephones clung to life a little longer, before mobile ownership became commonplace in the nineties – just as the internet was also beginning to blossom. First-generation mobile devices were not internet enabled, but once Wi-Fi, 3G and 4G mobile data breakthroughs arrived, all the conditions for the two technologies to be fused, and for phones to become indispensable personal super computers, had aligned. The consequences have been profound, permeating all aspects of life. In Western countries, unceasing connectivity now seems as natural as the air that we breathe, the virtual world melded into our physical world and always at our fingertips. The internet's contribution to education and work, as well as social interaction, has been immense. At its best, the net has become a phenomenally powerful force for good, for spreading knowledge and ideas throughout the world, enriching us all and strengthening communities. But for those whose digital life has lapsed into excess, is information overload a problem? A risk to health even? Robert Burton certainly thought so. Centuries before the digital revolution, the author of *Anatomy of Melancholy* was already concerned by the barrage of information reaching his eyes and ears:

> I hear new news every day, and those ordinary rumours of war, plagues, fires, inundations, thefts, murders, massacres, meteors, comets, spectrums, prodigies, apparitions, of towns taken, cities besieged in France, Germany, Turkey, Persia, Poland &c. daily musters and preparations, and such like, which these tempestuous times afford, battles fought, so many men slain, monomachies, shipwrecks, piracies, and sea-fights, peace, leagues, stratagems, and fresh alarms. A vast confusion of vows, wishes, actions, edicts, petitions, lawsuits, pleas, laws, proclamations, complaints, grievances, are daily brought to our ears.[2]

Burton was writing in the seventeenth century, a time when only word of mouth and an embryonic printed press existed to carry these unhappy tidings. Rolling news, most of it still bad, is now available to us around the clock and in real time – not only from the televised news but streamed across internet channels. The pleasure of checking our feeds can quickly turn to compulsion; why should I click this link to see how that fifteenth-seeded tennis player is getting on at the backwater open? Well, because *it's there*, so I can, and clicking it helps avoid other things I ought to be doing but don't really want to. The digital world is alive twenty-four-seven, and once we are connected it calls to us all the time, urging us to consume more and think less with scream-if-you-want-to-go-faster momentum. Opportunities for obsession and abstraction abound. It is perpetual overload. When computers are overloaded they crash, and something analogous may now be happening to our collective mental health.

Social Media

Looming clear of the infinite, pixelated mists of the digital ecosystem, social media has emerged to transform our lives, opening a gateway to a second, digital, life, but also to more scrutiny in the process. Use of the internet has climbed rapidly since the millennium. In the year 2000 just 25 per cent of UK households were connected to the internet; by 2019 that figure had soared to 93 per cent,[3] and use of social media has boomed in tandem. In 2007 just 22 per cent of the UK's population had one or more social media profiles, and by 2016 this figure had risen to 89 per cent.[4] Then, in 2019, the 'Internet access – households and individuals' report from the Office for National Statistics indicated that 98 per cent of sixteen-to-twenty-four-year-olds had used social media at least once in the last three months[5] – a virtual saturation. Many people, particularly the young, have accounts on several platforms, and though the data-collection practices of some have become notorious, a more prosaic concern for well-being is the sheer time demanded in servicing them, and the creeping addictiveness of it all. The magical combination of the internet grafted onto mobile technology has made digital life incessant. Humans are social animals, but for many, socialising online is now replacing socialising in person. We may have hundreds of connections on Facebook or LinkedIn, but do online interactions nourish the soul just the same? Is a childhood lived through social media really as good for well-being as one spent climbing trees or kicking a ball with friends? Have we become so preoccupied with photographing and cataloguing our lives online that we are now failing to truly live them? For many, catatonic scrolling has become a default state. But not all entertainment is leisure, and not all digital interaction is as richly fulfilling as socialising in the flesh. With online communication so dominant, we are now spending less time forging the real-world friendships that used to knit together physical communities. It has created a modern paradox whereby connectedness is rising hand in hand with isolation, loneliness growing as the world gets smaller.

Fear of Missing Out

The gap between the lives that most of us lead and the apparently gilded lifestyles we might see on social media is now more visible than ever before, and so feels bigger. This 'aspiration gap' has created a modern anxiety: Fear of Missing Out Syndrome, or FoMo. If we have nothing, and no knowledge of better, there is nothing to lose, and one source of anxiety is removed. Once we are granted a portal into the carefully curated showpiece worlds of others, seemingly leading idealised lives, it can throw our own perceived shortcomings into painfully sharp relief, rendering us akin to Dickensian urchins with noses pressed to the window, gazing in on a world we can't enter. In the twenty-first century we are saturated with choice, but that can, of itself, provoke anxiety if we become consumed by the fear that maybe we aren't making the right calls; that we are missing opportunities to live life to the fullest.

Emboldened behind the cover of avatars, a more deliberate form of distress is being inflicted by online trolls and cyberbullies. When people with contrasting views meet online the result is often immediate hostility, greater polarisation, and yet more digging in of already entrenched positions. The semi-detached medium and physical distancing making it too easy to bypass old-fashioned courtesy and rush straight to naked abuse. Now that social media is near ubiquitous, some users, children especially, have taken to maintaining an almost unceasing dialogue with one another. Such contact can be fulfilling, helping to grow and fortify new friendships, but this too can be abused. The age-old blight of bullying, once partly constrained by school hours, can feel relentless and inescapable in an age when bullies can intrude into time at home using social media. Direct messaging apps too can be problematic when used as vehicles for spreading hurtful images or content. Some 70 per cent of young people report having experienced some form of cyberbullying at least once, and 37 per cent say that they are suffering abuse on a frequent basis.[6] Misused technology has liberated the more pernicious aspect of human nature, always there, by circumventing natural checks that had hitherto denied it such reach and expression. This is a direct risk to mental health. Victims of bullying are known to be more likely to suffer depression and anxiety, to sleep poorly, and to self-harm.[7]

Digital Marketplaces

It is not just our social lives that have been transformed by online technologies but our experiences as workers and consumers too. The digital revolution and mature, globalised capitalism have coincided to spectacular effect, and with the powers of the digital world harnessed to the pursuit of profit, working patterns have evolved to take advantage of new possibilities for enhancing the productivity of labour. Emails in combination with smartphones have extended the reach of the office beyond the traditional nine-to-five. Without really knowing how we got here, many are now living for work rather than working to live. Can this be healthy? Is a working world of harassed individuals in the thrall of apparently inescapable symbiotic relationships with mobile devices really desirable?

The value of psychology, and especially psychoanalysis, has long been appreciated by economists, and by businesses wanting to get into the heads of customers. Macroeconomists concern themselves with the wealth of nations, the balance of payments, imports, exports, gross domestic product and pretty much anything else fairly described as *gross* by the same definition. But these grand measures are nothing but an accumulated view of thousands upon thousands of individual transactions going on all the time at the micro level. The subdiscipline of microeconomics, defined as the branch of economics that studies the behaviour of individuals and firms when making decisions about the allocation of scarce resources, is really an aspect of psychology. What is underlying these behaviours that, in aggregate, constitute what we call markets? In microeconomics, individuals deciding how to spend their household budgets are assumed to be rational, seeking to maximise their utility. But the science behind this boils down to the consumer choices made by many millions of normal, complex, flawed humans, according to their personal preferences. Do we book that two-week tour of Tobago? Or should we put the money towards that extension, and bimble on the beach at Blackpool instead? The green boots or the red shoes? All the decisions we take are of immense interest to firms seeking to pitch their products and price points according to preference curve models that help them understand how we balance what we want with what we are willing to pay for it. To them, unblemished serenity is not economically desirable. If we are satisfied with our lot, why rush out and buy the latest products? Why strive to optimise utility if utility is already optimised? In the consumerist world we are constantly encouraged to hunger for something. In consequence, firms and marketeers, their interests aligned with our wants, find an incentive to needle our security, whether with our appearance, lifestyle or something else, encouraging us always to push for something newer, faster, bigger or better to fix whatever shape of hole we *think* we have inside us.

Once this consumer psychology ran into the possibilities created by the digital revolution, things not previously commoditised rapidly became so. A transformational explosion of the consumer experience accompanied the onset of the digital age. Online shopping, banking and trading introduced fresh convenience into our lives, but in an unbound, pervasive form that corporations could have previously only dreamed of. Our exposure to marketing is no longer limited to pages in a magazine or the television advert breaks. Now it is personalised in the unrelenting attention economy. Sometimes we don't even know it is happening. Our personal data, click habits and the inferences they permit have become, of themselves, objects of trade. Prized by corporations eager to know what books we might read, what music we might want, and who might have overspent at Christmas and need a loan in January, all to better target their activities and maximise revenues. Occasionally this goes too far, when the insights harvested from our many 'likes' are improperly accessed or used, as was alleged with the Cambridge Analytica scandal of 2018.

In recent decades a wealth of inventive products has arisen to take advantage of these new online markets. But the addictive urge to have the digital world rush through our screens can bring real-life impacts on our relationships, our well-being, and ultimately our mental health. It is now easier than ever before to indulge weaknesses that may otherwise have remained dormant in the absence of easy opportunity. Those with a predisposition for betting, for instance, are no longer obliged even to stretch their legs and visit a high-street bookie, but can lay bets on almost anything, day or night, from anywhere using their smartphones. There's always something happening for us to bet on somewhere in a connected world. Temptations abound, but if you're going to swim with the sharks you better learn not to bleed.

Dating apps too are now big business. In America they are already the most common way new couples meet,[8] and the UK is heading in the same direction. With vast numbers now signed up, they present us with more potential matches than ever before – perhaps more than we can properly process. Does this devalue them? Might we be less inclined to overlook even minor flaws and devote time to working at a relationship now armies of potential replacements are available on tap, potentially just a click away from usurping that errant spouse who has left a wet towel on the floor, again? The architecture of many dating apps is heavily geared towards aesthetics, encouraging users to pass judgement on potential matches rapidly, and the risk is that this may trigger a short-term mating psychology, whereby we forge, abandon and switch relationships more casually than is good for us. Previous generations selected partners from a far narrower pool, limited by the circles travelled in their social and professional lives. The processing power required to evaluate potential partners remained within the capacity of the human brain. Today singletons are attempting to navigate an anchorless world of infinite 'just maybes', with heightened risks of loving not wisely, but too well.[9] There must be some trade-off between the benefits of extended choice that these apps provide and the risk of overload, ultimately diminishing the odds of finding a true meeting of minds, values and temperament that lasts the long haul. The architecture of some apps now even incorporates aspects of the reward structure beloved of the gambling industry, using algorithms that pull cutely on our striatum – the part of the brain that anticipates rewards, chasing down the dopamine rush released when we hit the jackpot. In this way the online dating industry has weaponised the addiction principle of providing unpredictable yet frequent hooks in its race to replace Cupid, who must surely be up there somewhere, strumming a harp and reflecting ruefully that his troubles with Psykhe were as nothing compared to all this.

Dating apps have only been in the mainstream for a little over a decade. What will be their long-term impact on our rubric of relationships, families and societal cohesiveness, particularly in conjunction with secularism and softening of faith nibbling at the same fabric? The traditional family unit is already declining in increasingly atomised societies. Monogamous marriage is not the only show in town. of course; other domestic arrangements are equally valid and can be just as conducive to our well-being. But it is generally recognised that a stable home life, in whatever form, provides not just economic benefits but comfort and security that can safeguard us against mental ill health. Stability and swipe culture are not natural bedfellows, and who can say where the digital world will sweep our dating habits, interpersonal relationships, and lifestyles from here?

The Digitally Excluded

At the opposite pole from those for whom life has become excessively digital are the 'digitally excluded'. Their plight is to find online participation either inaccessible or incompatible in a world that is coming to insist upon it. As with overuse, having no digital presence whatsoever can carry disadvantages. In the twenty-first century it can lead to isolation and increased difficulty managing the basic requirements of daily life. Governments and corporations are using 'nudge' tactics to shunt ever greater proportions of business onto the internet, everything from submitting self-assessment tax returns to booking GP appointments or renewing TV licences. Banks are actively engaged in an overt policy of closing branches and diverting transactions online, and some retailers and energy and insurance providers offer preferential rates reserved only for those buying online, all sending savings to their bottom line. This creates convenience for some but barriers for others. Digital is a great option, but a zeitgeist assumption that it should be the *only* option, even for accessing basic services, risks excluding a whole cohort of people who are unable or unwilling to follow the digital herd. Not everyone has the capacity to conduct vital aspects of their life online, and it is not a trivial proportion of our communities. The group includes some with disabilities, and some who lack the means to pay for internet access. These people should not be stereotyped as out-of-date or old, or asked to get with the times if doing so comes at the expense of their well-being.

Last of the Innocents?

If we could pause time and perform a digital cross-section of the Western population we would find a portrait of stark juxtaposition. The baby boomer generation now entering retirement encountered online life only in mature adulthood; their formative years were lived well before the social media age. Coming after them in the demographic are the people of generations X and Y, who may have used computers as children, but who reached maturity before the internet bloomed into widespread use. Following them are the millennials and generation Z, whose lives have been saturated in social media and mobile technology from their earliest memories. Humanity will soon reach a point where no one alive can remember a world without the internet. Those born before 1980 have been dubbed 'the last of the innocents', the final generation with lived experience of what it was to be human before the Digital Age. Once they are gone, no one will truly know what it was to experience the world at its former pace, save any who seek out an 'off-grid' lifestyle and who will likely be thought eccentric for doing so. No one will know the need to find ways of killing time, or be left with nothing to do but surrender to the void that nurtures flights of imagination, moments when we are alone with only our thoughts and interior selves. No one will remember what it was to have the time to stop and stare. When that moment arrives, what will we have lost? We cannot know.

Since the internet's beginnings the world has completed insufficient revolutions for us to be sure. The advances that got us here – mastery over electricity, the invention of computers, the rise of the World Wide Web – all accrued iteratively, step by step, each new invention a marginal contribution extending the frontier that bit further. When change depends on lots of little advances that span generations there is no grand design, no individual agent with control across the whole piece, no overarching clarity of direction. This partially organic characteristic of the arc of technological progress creates the possibility that some outcomes produced, as events accelerate and spiral, may not be desirable. The pace of digital developments is still picking up all the time. What will the implications of decisions taken in Silicon Valley today be for the mental health of tomorrow? That too we cannot know, nor can anyone in the valley. We are on a journey into virgin territory (although there may just be apps that can change all that). But scientific debate over whether sustained internet use has a damaging effect on the brain and on our mental health is well underway, with academics hungrily seeking hard evidence on the question. While prevalence of mental ill health has not altered appreciably at the whole population level in the historical blink of an eye for which data is available, anxiety and depression among the UK's young people is one substratum where levels have risen, and dramatically so – by almost 50 per cent since 2004.[10] This period directly coincides with the transition to present circumstances where 98 per cent of sixteen-to-twenty-four-year-olds in the UK use social networking sites regularly. These individuals belong to generation Z, the front-line digital natives who have never known a world without the internet. Evidence that the correlation between their increased internet use and increased rates of mental ill health may be causation not coincidence arrived in 2019, when *World Psychiatry* published the results of an international study concluding that excessive internet use produces 'acute and sustained alterations in specific areas of cognition',[11] suggesting that digital overuse does adversely impact cognitive functioning, attention span and memory.

Other big questions are coming over the hill. Our online life has created fresh vulnerability to corruption and to crimes that we have spent centuries learning to guard against. The *Magna Carta*, the elimination of rotten boroughs, and the achievement of universal suffrage in Britain, the Bill of Rights in the United States, and all subsequent defences against electoral fraud and political corruption were hard won and long in the making. Our shift to the nascent digital dimension of fake news, hacking, micro targeting, Twitter bots, and misinformation now imperils them in ways that could not have been foreseen. When the Nazi doctrine spread through Germany with alarming rapidity and found acceptance with unsettling ease, it was widely acknowledged that Joseph Goebbels' mastery of the media was vital to the process. Back then, the tools at his disposal were the print media, the wireless, and the spoken word. How much easier to achieve mass subversion with the uber-powered communications channels of modernity in the hands of a skilled manipulator? The impact of that on societal well-being cannot even be guessed at. Groupthink, the state that arises when independent thought is impaired by an overriding compulsion to conform at all costs to the majority view, finds fertile ground in the self-selecting, insular networks that can form online. Within their confines defences go up, humanity down, and rational thinking often ends up out of the window. Demonisation of the 'outgroup' – those taking opposing views – can easily result. Nietzsche's aphorism 'In individuals, insanity is rare; but in groups, parties, nations and epochs, it is the rule'[12] describes the effect. These are the same underlying dynamics Goebbels was exploiting, and which incubated the seventeenth-century witch craze in Salem. Collective hysteria liberated and writ large. We have our warnings from history. Today, it is often those with sincere wishes to be progressive who insist most vociferously on absolutist conformity to their narrative, which they intend to be libertarian and politically correct. Whatever good intentions might be motivating them, there are in reality few more fundamental suppressions of liberty than the suppression of free thought and free speech – and few more dangerous than insistence upon a single, mandated world view, particularly when that insistence is enforced through vilification of anyone who dares deviate from it. We must now find a way to walk the tightrope of constraining illegal and hateful content online and protecting hard-won liberal freedoms without resorting to reactionary measures that themselves infringe upon those very freedoms, sleepwalking into a culture of coercive conformity of the type Orwell warned of:

> Every record has been destroyed or falsified, every book rewritten, every picture has been repainted, every statue and street building has been renamed, every date has been altered. And the process is continuing day by day and minute by minute. History has stopped. Nothing exists except an endless present in which the Party is always right.[13]

Digital Horizons

In historical terms, the Digital Age is still taking its first breaths. We have opened a door and the future is rushing in, but it doesn't necessarily look like the future we were expecting. With the pace of change now so ferocious, regulation is inevitably playing catch-up and our digital technology may be starting to resemble an uncontrollable overlord rather than a servile automaton. A pause to cultivate the support structures that will allow us to navigate the digital world healthily, ameliorating the situations of those who can't, feels overdue. Structures needed to safeguard us against the risk of humanity's place in the digital future being reduced to that of a cork bobbing about in the ocean. No one is suggesting we should abandon modern technology, or that we could do so even if we wanted to; that genie is not just out of the bottle, it has vanished into the cloud, and the potential social benefits of modern technology are immense. It is not that we *have* a digital life that is the issue, but that we have not yet mastered the art of living it well. For the sake of human well-being, learning to do so must be a legislative priority.

In the globalised age, international cooperation will be required if there is to be any hope of controlling web-based behemoths whose products transcend national boundaries. In the meantime, one act that remains in the gift of any of us feeling overwhelmed is the simple step of voting with our feet and disconnecting more frequently. This is easier said than done when the whole world seems permanently online, but the fact that something has become locked into normality doesn't necessarily make it desirable. QWERTY is not the most efficient distribution of letters across a keyboard, but it was the first arrangement to gain popular acceptance, and so became locked in. We know now that other arrangements are easier to learn, but no manufacturer diverging from QWERTY could expect market success now that QWERTY is embedded as being what the great majority who *already have* learned now know and expect. A self-perpetuating cycle. Perhaps we only have all those social media accounts because everyone else has all those accounts, and so it must be the thing to do. Maybe spending our time online because we think there is nothing better to do is preventing us from finding better things to do. Maybe we are in the grip of a collective addiction, and need to consciously disrupt the cycle for the sake of our well-being.

Despite the extent of their importance initially being underappreciated, it is clear now that the innovations of Tomlinson and his fellow digital pioneers are transforming the world, touching the lives of almost everyone. Yet still we perceive only the tip of the digital iceberg. So what comes next? Another major shift in labour markets looks likely, where a constant state of flux may become the norm in the post-Covid world. Automation of routine manual labour has been happening since the first Industrial Revolution, but algorithms with the ability to learn are now bringing the same possibilities to the creative vocations. No longer is it just factory workers, check-out cashiers or taxi drivers at risk of being displaced by automatons and driverless cars; functions like drafting legal documents, making medical diagnoses and even architecture and design are coming within scope of learning technologies. If we are transitioning to a workless world the process could constitute a liberation, freeing up thousands of hours for many millions worldwide to spend enjoying family, travel, learning, leisure or anything else. But work can also be fulfilling, providing people with purpose in life and job satisfaction, and if our digital genius ever brings us to the point where humanity is able to dispense with it the leap will need to be carefully made, with a new basis for distributing income, wealth and resources found in the process.

So are we in the ascent to a digitally driven paradise? Or is humanity about to be consumed by a digital dystopia? It is a question that simultaneously excites and terrifies. The showdown between Frankenstein and his monster, between man and inexorably advancing machine, has long been a staple of science fiction. But generating ever more sophisticated machines is not the only possibility for science. The Turing Test of artificial sophistication judges machines according to their ability to imitate human intelligence, but instead of striving to make computers more intelligent, what if we used our technological knowledge to enhance our own minds, so that it is we who become more sophisticated? Then the Turing Test becomes a red herring, as man and machine advance together. One intriguing possibility is 'mind uploading'. This is the idea that once technology has progressed sufficiently, the brain could be scanned in fine detail, and all memories and even personality duplicated in digital form. This may sound like something that belongs alongside Frankenstein in the realm of fiction, but it is now also a subject of serious interest for some of the world's most eminent academics, like Princeton professor Michael Graziano, whose 2019 book *Rethinking Consciousness: A Scientific Theory of Subjective Experience* includes a landmark exploration of the possibility. And mind uploading is a possibility that needs no further Eureka moments or vaulting leaps of understanding to bring about, just iterative improvements in existing technologies along their current trajectories.

Would replication in perfect precision produce the breath of life? According to proponents of the theory, the result of a mind upload would be a divergent tree branch, a perfect consciousness replica existing in parallel with its real-world template. But unlike the biological original, this artificially created divergence would be potentially immortal, subject to its host cloud being maintained. The world that these copies inhabit would not necessarily remain a shadowland, detached from physical reality, but could interface with the biological world using digital mediums. Email, app-based direct messaging and video conferencing are already part of the twenty-first-century furniture, and leveraging the same infrastructure a whole plethora of jobs could be readily done by an intelligence resident in the cloud. Indeed, creative and strategic functions might even lend themselves more naturally to cloud-based workers who would be able to fuse more directly with the augmented processing power available there to accomplish the most complex, high-end tasks. For these reasons Graziano and other students of mind uploading argue that power would inevitably gravitate towards the cloud, with the biological world slowly relegated to the status of a training pen, a nursery in which the very young would learn, before shedding their chrysalis forms and making the ascent to the cloud, where the real work would begin with all that big data and symbiosis between human consciousness and machine memory available to process it. As yet there is no consensus within the scientific community about whether mind uploading will inevitably become part of our future, but if it does ever make the jump from science fiction it is a symbiosis that could elevate human cognitive potential beyond fatigue, possibly beyond all limitation. It could smash the glass ceiling that has historically limited machines too, by lending them the capacity for creative thought, and with it the opportunity to transcend their original programming.

We look back and speculate what the great names of past times would make of the world of today, people like Hippocrates, Descartes, Shakespeare, Churchill and Freud. Perhaps future generations won't have to wonder. Perhaps in years to come they might enjoy direct access to icons who, for us, are yet to come, but for them will have gone before, the essence of these future geniuses not merely preserved in passive afterlife but freed by technology to go on contributing to societies indefinitely, both the biological and the cloud.

Mind uploading is a tantalising prospect, apparently offering a means to shift the frontiers of human potential, and gifting us an eternity to explore its new scope. A scan of infinite granularity, shining a light into every corner of the mind, could finally pierce the mysteries that have long shrouded the workings of the brain. But mind uploading raises plenty of moral questions too, not least when it comes to mental health. Though we like to think we enjoy uncompromised free will, humans are not unlike machines already in the sense that we are 'programmed' in part by our genetic inheritance, and in part by our environments and experiences. It is this code that determines our thoughts, feelings and behaviours, making us who we are. In the act of cloning, people would be disaggregated and then reproduced in the cloud. Any aspects of the unique code we call 'us' but which we deem undesirable could be isolated in the process, raising the possibility that people could be freed from illness, disability, infirmity or even quirks of character in the rebuilding. Any hurtful memories could be likewise removed, the trauma instantly cauterised. But if humanity does make mind uploading a reality, exposing the mind's most minute operations, *should* we choose to exercise the power? Choose to isolate the code that causes mental ill health, and eliminate it in the upload? Go further perhaps and eliminate all negative thoughts, emotions or predispositions for envy, lust, or vice; attempting to create a more intelligent, super-tuned, super-capable version of our best selves? Would whatever was left after all this really still be *us*? Maybe somewhere in humanity's future the long-sought-after key to understanding the human soul is to be found, and ironically it just might be the tree of knowledge that ultimately paves the way to the Promised Land beyond our earthly world. Just possibly mind uploading might offer humanity the pathway to the sunlit paradise described in the creation myths of so many cultures, whether as Nirvana, Arcadia, Elysium, Jannah or Eden. Then again, perhaps things will work out like the last time humanity ate from the tree of knowledge, or the last time a regime sought to arbitrate which traits should be propagated, which eliminated, who should live and who should die. To determine what constitutes life worthy of life. Perhaps if we do ever achieve the technology needed to eternally preserve our 'best selves', free of inner turmoil, we would inevitably have to sacrifice something fundamental to our humanity in the bargain. Perhaps that will be the moment when *Homo sapiens* evolves into something else entirely. Then again, perhaps it's already happened. Maybe we are hardwired to the matrix already, and perhaps that's not even real steak either.

9

FOODS FOR THOUGHTS – HOLISTIC HEALTH

Mental health is an essential component of all health. In the World Health Organisation's constitution it is written that 'health is a state of complete physical, mental and social well-being and not merely the absence of disease or infirmity'.[1] Four hundred years after the ideological duel over mind and body had seemingly ended in victory for Cartesian dualism, the ideas of Descartes are losing their lustre, and the pendulum of popularity is swinging back towards Spinoza. The purely biological construction of health pathology that long held sway is giving way to an appreciation that the condition of our minds has a profound impact on our bodies and vice versa, debunking the notion that physical and mental health are distinct by materiality. We now know that they are conjoined, and that human nature, entire and whole and imperfect, is dangerously misunderstood when we compartmentalise physical and mental health as separate.

Physical and Mental Health

Physical health problems inevitably carry psychological implications, particularly serious or long-term conditions like cancer, diabetes, COPD and others that may bring functional impairments necessitating major adaptations or lifestyle changes. Receiving such a serious diagnosis is an obvious blow, and lack of attention to the psychological dimension of such conditions may leave people less able to make the lifestyle adjustments required of them. Conversely, poor mental health is associated with higher rates of problematic alcoholism, drug use and smoking, as well as diminished employment prospects – all recognised risk factors for a broad range of physical health issues.[2] This awakening to mind/body interconnectedness did not happen overnight, and while it was spreading, so too the importance of social determinants of health was also beginning to register, encompassing factors such as isolation, loneliness, poverty, abuse and neglect. Steadily, a holistic, 'biopsychosocial model' that considers health as a product of biological, psychological and social forces in combination has become orthodox.

In a 2018 article for the *Independent* I described the situation of the growing numbers of people who today find themselves in circumstances where multiple, interrelated problems of all these types are crowding upon them simultaneously. Many end up presenting to the NHS with health issues, but may also be in independent contact with agencies helping with their finances, their housing needs, addictions or the criminal justice system. The main cause of their distress is often unclear, as is whether they really have a health condition by conventional definitions at all. Is this person's mood low because they aren't sleeping, or is it because they are drinking every night? Is work stress causing this drinking, or is the drinking creating problems with sleep and work that are perhaps now growing so serious the individual fears losing their job altogether, and with it the roof over their head? The stress of all this may be threatening to stop them functioning *at all*, making whole-life collapse a real possibility, and naturally causing them to drink all the more. Is this spiral fuelling their physical and mental health issues? Or is it really the health issues at the root of these lifestyle choices? *When sorrows come, they come not single spies, but in battalions,*[3] and it is no coincidence; the relationships are symbiotic and circular.

Complex, biopsychosocial factors such as these – in other words, the daily experiences of millions of ordinary people – span the traditional thresholds of health and social care. No one professional has hold of the whole thread, and it is difficult to identify where the thread begins. Our physical health, diets and sleep patterns, our social and working lives, our family and economic circumstances and our mental health are all interrelated. The forces exerted are not one-way; there is multi-directional interplay at work. Trying to neatly unpick all this to think of our mental health in isolation is like trying to unscramble an omelette. While this biopsychosocial understanding of humanity and health has now achieved broad acceptance, the talk we talk in academic and professional circles has yet to translate fully into walking the walk. As well as dying hard, old habits leave a legacy, and one hangover from our Cartesian thinking has been a health system where mental and physical services remain commissioned and delivered largely separately. It is not quite 'never the twain shall meet',[4] but the twain are nodding acquaintances at most.

The National Health Service

Although we often think of the National Health Service as a thing – albeit a hulking, monolithic thing – it is in fact a series of things, a great multitude of separate legal entities, or NHS trusts, all engaged in one aspect or another of the commissioning, delivery and oversight of health and health-related services. Each has individual agendas, priorities, remits and responsibilities which, it is hoped, add up to good effect in the round. National strategy imposes some overarching commonality of direction, but the healthcare system is not – and never could be given its size – a perfectly synchronised machine with every cog connected to every wheel.

The National Health Service and Community Care Act of 1990 and National Health Service Act of 2006 established then consolidated NHS trusts as a central component of government attempts to decentralise control over healthcare, vesting authority in de facto public corporations responsible for health within their particular region. But division of responsibility is not purely regional. Some functions, deemed specialised, were stripped out and entrusted to another layer of separate NHS entities, so that there may in fact be several trusts involved in overlapping aspects of healthcare in any given locality. A hospital trust, for example, may be charged with looking after the acute healthcare needs of a city, but relies upon the performance of a separately constituted ambulance trust to transport emergency cases into its wards. And every locality is also served by its own mental health trust, another field deemed to require separate arrangements, exactly along the old Cartesian fissure. This macro system design does not, of itself, preclude the possibility of complementary coworking across the whole piece – joined-up centres of excellence each bringing their own specialisms to the greater effort. But in practice this is logistically difficult to deliver, especially when financial pressures bite. Each separate legal entity has its own funding streams and individual budget to protect. So in times of austerity, and when a patient's journey may touch several NHS trusts, each may discover perverse incentives to behave in ways unthinkable in a system designed on different lines. When an organisation finds its budget overspent and the pressure on, what unconscious vacillations might arise in well-intentioned but exhausted staff to prejudice decision making? Whose responsibility is the next patient in line? Can their complex, nuanced needs really be best met by us, with our waiting lists backing up out of the door, and resources already stretched as they are? Or does this look like someone whose needs might be better met by the other lot? When the multifaceted, biopsychosocial image of many people's cases is overlaid like a transparency onto our health system's rigid structural lines, scope for honest doubt often remains.

The ideal solution is collaborative, integrated care accompanied by decision making separated from, and blind to, all resourcing considerations. But further barriers to joined-up working are found in the vast, murky depths of excess bureaucracy and governance, something large public organisations are particularly prone to. On these rocks many collaborative ambitions have foundered, broken apart by the abstruse bureaucracy that spawns when NHS organisations seek to concert their efforts while simultaneously watching their own backs. Esoteric red tape and impenetrable legalese can torpedo whole projects. Commencing on the commencement date, the interpretation of all singular words shall be importing the plural and the vice versa, particularly but not limited to delay, decay, thumb twiddling and bemiring in the be-mud, before terminating on the termination date providing always that with the ball pitched outside the stumps, the batsman was playing a shot, and no one is in any way liable for anything. Or as Sir Humphrey expounded on a similar theme:

> There is a real dilemma here. In that, while it has been government policy to regard policy as a responsibility of Ministers and administration as a responsibility of Officials, the questions of administrative policy can cause confusion between the policy of administration and the administration of policy, especially when responsibility for the administration of the policy of administration conflicts, or overlaps with, responsibility for the policy of the administration of policy.[5]

Faced with verbiage like that, what is a well-intentioned organisation to do? Perhaps employ an army of consultant legal experts to keep their noses clean, paying them the money that would have gone on collaborating in the first place, so that change becomes unaffordable anyway, and things carry on pretty much as before? Any compromise results that do issue forth risk being badly mutilated – the blueprint for a camel. In this way bureaucracy interferes with integrated care, and people may be lost down cracks in the system. But for this to happen there must be cracks in the first place. When systems minimise interfaces, cohesive care always follows more naturally, and self-reported patient experience is uniformly smoother and more satisfactory. For these reasons reaching a better state of joined-up care has been a long-standing holy grail in health and social care services, but making things work in the real world has proved difficult. Few policy aspirations have received so much promotion yet translated into so little in the way of practical results. Beyond problems at the level of interface between different NHS bodies, meaningful connectivity has been hampered by a system not designed to accommodate the intrinsic interplay between health and those 'whole-life' social factors. NHS services deliver their part of the whole, local authorities theirs, and justice and employment services theirs too, while charities often serve an important but independent function trying to plug gaps in the middle. Workers on the ground try to join dots and help people as best they can, but basic expedients are still missing. In an always-on digital world our health and social care services remain conspicuously disconnected, lacking common IT systems or agreed protocols for sharing valuable information. Opportunities to improve joined-up working are too often sacrificed to excessively circumspect interpretations of patient confidentiality and data protection rules – rules that were originally intended to ensure that patient data *is* available to those who have a legitimate need to know it, as much as to lock it down from inappropriate disclosure to those who don't.

There is a similarly striking divergence between the physical and the psychological in the institutions where our modern-day medics receive their training before being freed to wield stethoscopes in anger in the wild. With the right choices (or wrong ones, depending on your perspective), it is possible for newly qualified doctors to emerge blinking into the world with only a rudimentary proportion of their training spent studying mental health before they take up their role as the GP gatekeepers to their locality's care pathways for the next forty or fifty years. *Bringing Together Physical and Mental Health: A New Frontier for Integrated Care*, a 2016 report by the King's Fund, a charity and research organisation working to improve health and care in England, called for

> new approaches to training and development ... to create a workforce able to support integration of mental and physical health. This has significant implications for professional education; all educational curricula need to have a sufficient common foundation in both physical and mental health.[6]

This looks like the low-hanging fruit of an easy win in the context of our present systems.

Addictions

Underestimating the links between our physicality and psychology doesn't just hamstring the system treating mental health issues after problems develop; it also hampers prevention if we take insufficient account of those links when making the many lifestyle choices that influence our mental health and our chances of developing problematic issues in the first place. The stresses associated with modern life have given rise to a slew of mechanisms for coping with them; some are new, others are as old as the hills.

Seeking consolation at the bottom of a bottle is one such method. The British have a long and loving relationship with alcohol. The tradition of monastic brewing in England goes back centuries, and Scotland is as closely associated with beautiful whisky as it is stunning forests and lochs. Occasionally the relationship gets so close as to provoke concerns. A 'gin craze' in the early eighteenth century had handwringers convinced that gin houses, popular dens for the indulgence of 'mother's ruin', were corruptive and would surely unhinge society. There followed numerous Acts of Parliament designed to curb the affordability and popularity of grain-based alcoholic drinks. Across the Atlantic, the Eighteenth Amendment to the United States Constitution introduced a thirteen-year period of prohibition from 1920 as America struggled to reconcile the Temperance movement's puritanism with the individual's freedom to sink a skinful if they so desired. Prohibition gave rise to a black market ripe for exploitation by bootleggers like Al Capone, and left millions feeling short measured before the passage of the Twenty-First Amendment reversed it in 1933.

In the twenty-first century concerns are again heightened that self-medicating with alcohol is becoming dangerously routine for a whole new generation of people. But today's cohort have a fresh aesthetic – no longer just the dishevelled, hard drinkers of cliché, but a more gender-balanced, often employed, and often high-functioning group of professionals who have adopted wine o'clock as their coping mechanism – a fixed-point release that keeps everything else turning around it. An occasional glass surely remains one of life's pleasures, but dispatching a whole bottle of Châteauneuf-du-Pape in one sitting every evening will do nothing good for the liver, bank balance or mood. When alcohol takes hold to become an indispensable crutch for getting from day to day it is a tocsin that something is out of kilter. Insidiously and by degrees consumption that might have felt controllable bleeds into addiction, and the risks to health edge higher. People seeking to escape their unhappiness may indeed find temporary release the night before, but life hits all the harder the morning after, when the shame-filled hangover leaves them feeling only more hopeless. The devil is then in the act of trying to break the cycle. While judgmental attitudes towards mental health issues in general are now encountered less frequently, people often remain quick to judge the alcoholic, missing the despairing human behind the visible behaviour of the addict.

Self-medicating can carry even greater risks when drugs and not alcohol, or perhaps some combination of both, are the agents used to relieve stress. The post-industrial supply chain advancements that transformed legitimate commerce had the same effect upon black markets too, making drugs available to many who would previously have had no access. The 'lights of perverted science'[7] even created new drugs that *could not* have existed, let alone have been affordable at scale to most people, in past centuries. An underground market has spawned where consumers can quickly find themselves descending the slippery slope to addiction, whether succumbing to the pernicious effects of lower-classification drugs or the nakedly brutal devastations of newer, chemically manufactured Class As – steroids on steroids. Excess alcohol or drug use also invites side effects, including the disturbed circadian rhythm that results when stimulants are introduced to the body. Good sleep is vital to our ability to regulate our biological systems and our mental health, something even the comic creations of P. G. Wodehouse acknowledged:

'One of the Georges,' said Psmith, 'I forget which, once said that a certain number of hours' sleep a day – I cannot recall for the moment how many – made a man something, which for the time being has slipped my memory. However, there you are. I've given you the main idea of the thing; and a German doctor says that early rising causes insanity.'[8]

The relationship between mental health and sleep is actually even more nuanced than the erudite Psmith imagines. As with all aspects of our physical and mental health, cause and effect is a two-way street, and circular dependencies are at work. Mental ill health, particularly anxiety, can disrupt our ability to fall and stay asleep, and we are all familiar with the cognitive sluggishness that results. Similarly, lack

of sleep can cause poor mental health. Sleep passes not as
a single state but in cycles, typically of between 60 and
120 minutes in duration. We need to have been asleep for
roughly 90 minutes before entering Rapid Eye Movement
(REM) sleep, and so waking frequently through the night
can cause us to miss out on this vital state. It is during REM
sleep that our most vivid dreams occur, as our brain is busy
processing emotions and experiences. As a result, achieving
REM sleep in good quantities is an essential precondition
for good mental health, but here again our nocturnal routine
is another sphere where digital modernity has introduced
a new dynamic. Millions now sleep with mobiles charging
on the bedside table, perhaps setting an app to wake them
in place of the traditional alarm. After lights out, millions
too succumb to the temptation to reach for their phones to
send that overlooked email, make a note about a forgotten
job, check their social media, perhaps even trawl the net for
apps to help beat insomnia, or to do something else equally
stimulating to the brain. The Greeks thought that their god
of sleep, Hypnos, had a claim over half of their lives, but for
most today the idea of a solid twelve hours is simply not an
option. We are getting significantly less sleep than we used
to,[9] and our body clocks aren't built for it.

Foods for Thoughts

Despite the fundamental function of sleep, when it
comes to finding the blend of social and lifestyle factors
that maximises our prospects for good mental health,
nothing tips the scales like our diet. In 1943, Abraham
Maslow listed food as one of the fundamental building

blocks of human motivation in his famed Hierarchy of Needs.[10] In order of progression, the full suite of criteria is: physiological well-being; safety; love and belonging; esteem; and self-actualisation.[11] We need the most basic foundations – sufficient physical security and freedom from immediate threat, somewhere to live and something to eat – before we can aspire to overlaying mental well-being and self-fulfilment upon this base. For those without these foundations securely in place, there is little hope of achieving upper-level contentment without first plugging the gaps. In this, Maslow pinpointed why homelessness, joblessness and the attendant uncertainties of each are such serious impediments to good mental health, and by implication why mental health services function best when they escape commissioning silos to work in concert with colleagues in physical health, housing, education and employment. The thinking also reinforces the fundamental importance of diet. We are what we eat, as the maxim goes, so it is no surprise that what we choose to put in our bodies influences how we feel. This might seem an obvious truth, but it was largely overlooked down the centuries of dualist thinking, when the concept of our bodies and minds as an integrated system was underappreciated. The typical Western dietary intake has changed markedly in recent decades. New technologies have found a raft of applications in the food industry, and the fruits of modern science are fuller, shapelier, and more liberally doused in fertilizer than ever before. Louis Pasteur's innovation with the thermal processing of milk, removing potentially harmful microorganisms and extending its shelf life, was a glorious example of applied science – an unqualified success that improved both food safety and food availability and has been practised for 160 years. It was one of many nineteenth- and twentieth-century breakthroughs that collectively delivered a substantial outward shift in the agricultural production possibility frontier, improving the scope and economic viability of agriculture and ultimately facilitating our modern mass-production techniques.

This uplift in capacity has been of immeasurable value in the effort to feed the world's rapidly growing population. With population growth showing no signs of slowing, and in an age when concerns over our climate and sustainability are also now intensifying, fresh technological breakthroughs may yet prove the best hope for sustaining humanity. To date, though, progressions in food technology have not been uniformly positive. The modern food industry is cutthroat like any other. For producers, the guiding market paradigm is not to maximise the health of end consumers but to optimise the economic efficiency of their output – achieving the greatest yield from production investment possible within the constraints of regulatory law. In consequence, practices like injecting growth hormones into livestock and 'reclaiming' meat have become common, allowing producers to squeeze a few more burgers off the production line and onto the bottom line. Injecting butchered poultry with water to bulk volume and create a plump, attractive aesthetic for consumers is another popular tactic. It may not be directly harmful – unless you're the chicken, of course – but does dilute the nutrition-by-volume value of our food intake.

The food industry now runs with 'just in time' supply chain efficiency with only a relatively small proportion of the population engaged in the production process. Most people have no input in supply chains besides appearing as end consumers, visiting supermarkets or awaiting home delivery of the neatly packaged staples rolling off production lines. Processed food has transformed the twenty-first-century diet. It is a diet that is no longer reliant on whole food consumption, as was the case with most of our ancestors, but now incorporates a growing proportion of 'junk' food, with the poorest communities particularly high consumers. Additives, preservatives and emulsifiers are commonplace in the many millions of prepared meals consumed each year, along with extra salt and sugar that makes it hard for people to track their intake. Is this merely a natural product of leaps in food technology that just happens to have coincided with the suggested modern mental health crisis? Or is causal interplay at work? After all, the food intake of many would have been unhealthy or inadequate before the arrival of processed foods.

For generations past, dietary options would have been constrained by economic means and, before extensive trade networks grew up, restricted to whatever could be grown locally or transported short distances before the food spoiled – and then only in whatever quantities the season's harvest permitted. These were people for whom living off the land meant the land beneath their feet. But although the diets of some may have been perilously constrained, they were at least constrained to whole foods. Go back far enough and even sugar and salt, beyond amounts naturally occurring, were rare in most diets. Sugar was considered a 'fine spice', and was prohibitively expensive for ordinarily people until bulk production in New World plantations began to drive prices down from the early eighteenth century. Salt too, though used for centuries for food preservation, was not the cheap, widely accessible commodity it is today. When viable deposits were found, whole towns sprang up to exploit them – the 'wich' in Nantwich, Northwich, Droitwich and others denoting their historic association with salt. Further afield wars were fought over salt trading routes and the taxes levied on them. So for most of human history, dietary intake, of whatever composition individual circumstances did or didn't permit, would at least have been relatively free of additives, artificial substances and excess salt and sugar – two of the substances most injurious to both waistlines and well-being when consumed in excess.

Our brains operate best on high-quality fuel, foods that deliver vitamins, minerals, nutrition and nourishment. Conversely, low-grade fuel, as might be obtained from diets heavy in processed foods, refined sugars or unhealthy levels of salt, correlates with diminished mental functioning and worsening of mood. Because diet is one aspect of life that has changed so markedly in recent generations, it is a sphere of life that deserves serious attention in an inquiry into a hypothesised deterioration of our collective mental health. And academic studies on the link between food and mood have found that incidence of depression among people consuming a typical, modern Western diet may be as much as 25 per cent higher in comparison with people sustaining themselves on a traditional 'Mediterranean' diet such as was common in the West before industrialisation[12] – one rich in whole foods, whole grains, vegetables, fish and fruit and near devoid of processed foods and artificial additives. Other studies have found that less healthy diets also correlate with a reduction in size of the brain's left hippocampus, the region associated with emotional regulation.[13] So there is growing evidence that our modern Western diet *is* influencing our mood, and may be another ingredient fuelling any modern mental health epidemic.

The trend towards less healthy diets has been amplified by our pervasive digital technology finding creative ways to fuse with the food industry. A raft of digital fast-food delivery services have sprung up to contribute their own dubious added value to the food industry landscape, offering temptations for time-poor diners. These services have knitted together two possibilities of the modern world – app-based technology and the gig economy – which now elbow their way into a middleman space in supply chains, linking consumers with food outlets (mostly fast-food outlets) via putatively self-employed delivery drivers. Do these apps make unhealthy choices too easy? Low-cost, low-nutrition, low-effort options may be creating a vicious circle, reinforcing both poor diets and sedentary lifestyles, and with a convenience that has seen demand balloon.

Beyond the influence diet exerts over our mood is the situation that arises when the relationship with food becomes the *primary cause* of a very specific health issue – as is the reality for people suffering with bulimia or anorexia. Body dysmorphic disorder (BDD), a preoccupation with one or more perceived bodily flaws, is another diagnosis often comorbid with eating disorders, but which is distinct in its own right. BDD is a condition particularly sensitive to the forces of the digital age, and the pressure to look good that can accompany life on social media. BDD was officially recognised in the third edition of the *Diagnostic and Statistical Manual of Mental Disorders* in 1980, and though it must have existed before then the opportunities for sufferers to plumb its miserable depths can have been nothing compared to today. Along with 'Fear of Missing Out Syndrome', which has jumped from the Urban Dictionary to *the Oxford English Dictionary* but has yet to make the *DSM*, BDD is surely a strong candidate for a disorder that the modern world can legitimately be said to have pushed into epidemic. The massive success of image-based social media, thriving on a model of taking, editing, posting and reacting to selfie after selfie after selfie, has created unprecedented pressure on users to focus on the superficial. In this goldfish-bowl culture insecurities can quickly become obsessions, and this may be a factor triggering BDD and its spread.[14]

Environmental Woes

There is another frontier to holistic health that feels like shifting the goalposts today, but which may become normalised in the fullness of time. As we increasingly recognise the importance of diet to mental health, and take ever greater interest in the agricultural supply chains that sustain us, we are learning once more to care more about the food we eat. Maybe we will also come to care more *for* the food we eat. Perhaps we are on the trajectory to a new method of measuring well-being where it will be counted at supra-species granularity, so that all life matters in the reckoning.

Populations of mammals, birds, fish, reptiles, and amphibians have, on average, declined by 60 per cent since 1970,[15] and the current rate of species extinction is estimated to be anywhere between 100 to 1,000 times higher than the background rate – the standard extinction rate through history before human activity became a prominent contributory factor.[16] The tragedy of these statistics rivals the 'one in four' prevalence of mental ill health, and the two are not unrelated. The prospects for planet earth matter to our mental health. Maslow's Hierarchy of Needs deals at the micro level of the individual human soul, but if we visualise a macro equivalent for the human race then the security of a safe, sustainable planet to live on must be the first rung of primary importance. If the planet is denuded of biodiversity, its oceans depleted, forests degraded, animals exploited and the climate thrown into unpredictable convulsions, the biological balance we depend on collapses into uncertainty. Conserving nature is an investment in conserving ourselves. We need a green industrial revolution, as transformative as the first, to usher in a raft of clean, low-carbon sources of power and technology that will allow us to maintain not just our new-found technologically enabled living standards, but also planet earth itself, and our very existence upon it.

Sat like a Russian doll within this planetary problem is the issue of industrial farming. Tens of billions of sentient lives are now lived and ended on production lines. Animal life lived briefly, purely in service of the food industry. It is a life grotesquely at odds with the evolutionary psychology of these animals with their ancient instincts rooted in a free way of life – a parallel with active *Homo sapiens* suddenly finding themselves cloistered away in offices pursuing unnaturally sedentary lifestyles, only with an abattoir and not a glass of red to end the day. The idea that humans will need to eat less meat in future is becoming mainstream as concerns about climate change heighten. Whatever quantum farming of the future operates at, there can be no excuse for cruelty remaining built into the design of its industrial processes. As of today, outright abuse is still commonly perpetrated beneath the noses of Western populations believing that they live in enlightened societies with robust animal rights measures protected in law. The common practice of separating newborn calves, social animals, from their mothers to maximise potential for humans to exploit their milk yield is one such outrage. Another is the fate of animals caged in crushingly restrictive environments, as is the case for billions of battery chickens. For these reasons industrial farming has been called the biggest crime in history,[17] causing more suffering than all wars combined. As Peter Singer framed it in his seminal book *Animal Liberation: A New Ethics for Our Treatment of Animals*, 'Pain is pain, and the importance of preventing unnecessary pain and suffering does not diminish because the being that suffers is not a member of our own species.'[18]

Thankfully, the news is not all bad. The same technology that infiltrated food production processes so successfully remains at work finding new applications. It is poised to revolutionise diets yet again. We have witnessed the birth of the lab-grown fake meat industry, and as the range of plant-based alternatives continues to rise, production costs falling all the while, both the need and the justification for eating meat in large quantities will continue to diminish. Organic, free-range and ethical foods have been growing in popularity, complementing a resurgent fashion for more traditional, whole food diets. Maybe this will boost our future mental health, and maybe it won't only be human mental health that benefits. In centuries to come perhaps every living soul, human or animal, will be cherished as a bearer of inherent grace, and the cause of animal welfare will leave the political fringe to become accepted wisdom. Perhaps we can dream of one day reaching the heights of civilisation where all animal exploitation and cruelty is unthinkable, and will seem as outdated to our descendants as slavery does to modern sensibilities – barbarity confined to the history books. Maybe when that happens, when all lives truly matter, we will have earned the favours of providence, and helping the world in this way we may discover that we have lifted the weight of it from our own shoulders in the process, drawing the sting from our modern epidemic.

10

PARITY OF ESTEEM – THE CASE
FOR PUBLIC INVESTMENT, AND THE
POLICY RESPONSE

Moral and Economic Arguments
From the World Health Organisation and the *Global Burden of Disease* reports produced by the Institute for Health Metrics and Evaluation in Washington to data from the Office of National Statistics, the Department of Health and NHS England at home, respected sources the world over have supplied a wealth of information about the reach of mental ill health today. Right now, 971 million people are thought to be coping with mental illness worldwide.[1] Just under 300 million are suffering with anxiety,[2] and another 250 million with a depressive condition.[3] In the UK, one in four of the population will experience a mental health problem in the course of any given year,[4] one in six at any given time,[5] and seventeen people die by their own hand

each day.[6] These are a few among a barrage of available facts that offer all the statistics we could want on mental ill health but add little to our understanding of what is being done about it.

The moral case for public investment in mental health services does not rely on statistics. Once it is accepted that depression, anxiety and all the rest cause real pain, the case is made. There is an obvious moral imperative to alleviate suffering wherever possible so that everyone has the chance to live their best life. This prize glistens uppermost, but a defining premise of economics is that resources are scarce. With so many people suffering, the scale of need is immense. Somewhere the path of good intentions must run into the roadblock of financial pragmatism, and difficult choices must be made.

Most Western societies have allocated at least some public funding to mental health services for a long time. But traditionally expenditure was limited to provision for the most serious cases – maintaining the asylums as an investment of last resort, to cloister away those whose continued liberty was deemed an unacceptable risk to the public. Beyond this, mild to moderate mental issues typically went ignored. Through the long heyday of institutionalisation, vast sums were spent interning the acutely unwell, while people with more common problems like anxiety and depression were largely left to their own devices. Ignoring the many and focussing on the few in this way was unhelpful to both – and, it turns out, to the Exchequer. This is because public investment in community therapies, to help people before they reach crisis point, is a classic case of spend to save. Every dollar, pound, or euro of state money spent on primary care mental health services has the potential to save many times that in other sectors reliant on the public purse. Opportunities to intervene before mild issues turn to moderate, and moderate to severe, are opportunities for diversionary bud nipping – a chance *not* to spend money managing people in hospitals down the line. On top of these savings, mental ill health is now the biggest cause of lost working days in the UK – some 12.8 million in 2018/19.[7] An economy is better served by a healthy, productive workforce than one characterised by anxiety and stress. Unresolved mental health issues cause sickness absence, loss of productivity and high staff turnover, and both employers and the state bear the associated costs once they hit the bottom line. By making therapy available on the NHS early, the state can intervene *before* problems spiral to the point where someone is no longer able to hold down a job, before they become dependent on the benefit system or turn to alcohol or drugs to cope, and before they are forced to present at an emergency ward because there is nothing else there for them. In any society that spends public money on social security, on public health services, and on law enforcement agencies to serve, protect and keep the peace, it makes obvious political and economic sense to get upstream of preventable demand on these services wherever possible. In this way, the state finds alignment of its interests in doing the right thing for the individual citizen with its economic interests, and so intuitively it feels that the financial arguments for public investment in mental health ought to be no less compelling than the moral ones.

Nevertheless, proving this economic argument is a different matter; calculating the net financial impact of intervening is anything but straightforward. Quantifying the increased productivity and tax yields available when people remain well, the value of potential savings across myriad public services in scenarios where people never need them, and weighing that against the costs of the interventions needed to bring the savings about is formidably complex as an academic exercise. In the real world, where many people endure psychological issues without seeking help and so exist beyond the bandwidth of official statistics, putting an all-inclusive pounds-and-pence figure to the national costs of mental ill health becomes nigh on impossible. Fortunately, NHS England made a stab at it anyway. Their figures are staggering. The *NHS Five Year Forward View for Mental Health* estimates the annual cost of mental illness to the UK economy at £105 billion a year.[8] Another striking claim is that mental health problems now represent the biggest single cause of disability in the UK.[9] The greatest opportunity for savings is thought to be the opportunity to divert people whose issues are primarily psychological away from accident and emergency departments, and the attentions of the police. Figures published in 2018 by Her Majesty's Inspectorate of Constabulary and Fire & Rescue Services suggest that the Metropolitan Police receive one call every four minutes about a mental health concern,[10] and that the cost of taking these calls is £70,000 per annum.[11] And this is just the sum spent answering the calls, before any costs are incurred through officers responding. The Met is one of more than forty police forces in the UK, and policing is just one public service among many. The most striking thing about these figures is that they are only the tip of a very big financial iceberg.

There is evidently much to play for, and with financial prizes so large in the offing the Exchequer's bean counters have taken notice. Recognition of the potential for economic gains was enshrined in *No Health without Mental Health* – the 2011 cross-governmental mental health strategy – and the Parity of Esteem agenda, the flagship policy championed by Minister for Care and Support Sir Norman Lamb to help mental health 'level up' and become equal in status with physical health. The Health and Social Care Act of 2012 then imposed a legal obligation on NHS organisations to deliver parity of esteem between physical and mental health by 2020. Though that deadline came and went with much distance still to be travelled, aiming for the stars sometimes reaches the moon, and it was at least a twenty-twenty vision of great clarity.

Improving Access to Psychological Therapies (IAPT)

Launched in 2007, the national Improving Access to Psychological Therapies (IAPT) programme was the Department of Health's chosen vehicle for bringing these ambitions into reality. IAPT is focussed on treating the mild to moderate conditions that fall short of crisis but constitute the great bulk of mental ill health prevalence. Back in 2004, the National Institution for Health and Care Excellence (NICE) conducted a first principles review of the evidence base for the effectiveness of different interventions used to treat depression and anxiety disorders. It concluded that cognitive behavioural therapy (CBT) was an effective first-line treatment but noted that it was simply not available in anything like the quantities needed to satisfy the great unmet need in our communities. The core objective of the subsequent IAPT programme was to rapidly uplift national capacity of talking therapists, primarily cognitive behavioural therapists but also clinicians trained in other modalities appropriate for primary care. Agreement to the investment was predicated on an expectation that this new model therapeutic army, once trained and into the shires, would be the mechanism for tapping into those vast potential savings available, and so the IAPT programme would eventually pay for itself – and then some.

To fund the programme, central government provided local NHS commissioning bodies with ringfenced money to mobilise the new IAPT services in their areas. An accompanying requirement to spend it raising their capacity of talking therapists so it was equal to treating at least 15 per cent of local need was also handed down. This prevalence benchmark was otherwise referred to as the Access Target, and all NHS providers would be measured against it. IAPT services would be characterised by a high-volume, fast-throughput philosophy, with very large numbers of people receiving a focussed series of therapy sessions, typically provided once a week over a short period of successive weeks, before being discharged. By these methods 'patient flow' would be maintained, waiting lists avoided, and people with mild to moderate needs who could still benefit from an injection of timely support would receive it, in large numbers, before their conditions could worsen. These endeavours were complemented by funding flowed through Health Education England and spent in conjunction with universities to train the workforce that would become the foot soldiers of the IAPT services, delivering talking therapies at an unprecedented scale.

IAPT was an ambitious policy, and the large sums spent launching and sustaining it meant that transparent measures were needed to gauge its success. Both in terms of delivering its financial objectives, for which such hopes were held, and the clinical outcomes achieved for people using the services. But how to measure the impact of therapy on mental health when mental health is largely unseen? In IAPT services this old obstacle was circumvented by routine use of standardised clinical questionnaires, completed by patients at the start of their therapy, the end, and at every session falling between. A series of questions covering service users' sleep, energy, perceptions of self-worth and whether they have suicidal thoughts were routinely asked, with each question having several possible answers, and each answer having a numerical score attached. Summing the values generated offers IAPT clinicians a numerical proxy for the degree of psychological distress present in every service user they encounter, and because the questionnaires are used every time a patient sees a therapist, progress can be tracked across a course of therapy. The data provided is then used to inform the ongoing conduct of case care for individuals, and also permits the service's clinical performance to be evaluated in aggregate. Used widely nationwide since 2008, the questionnaires also help minimise subjectivity in the act of diagnosis.

With numerical scores attached to mental distress it became possible to set a bar, beyond which any questionnaire responses would be deemed to have met the clinical threshold for depression or for anxiety. It remains an imperfect method reliant on self-reported data, but with the same questionnaires mandated nationally it has at least provided a standardised benchmark, and a consistent, evidence-based attempt to address the old conundrum of how the intangible can be grasped. Armed with these diagnostic questionnaires and a data-driven mantra of 'measure, evidence and improve', the new IAPT services provided a 'stepped care' clinical model, meaning that the least resource-intensive therapy likely to benefit each patient is offered first. This is another founding principle of the model, designed to spread the therapeutic resources available as far as possible into their local communities, teeming with millions who could benefit from it. Combining these ingredients within the structure of a national programme, IAPT was a serious and organised attempt to get to grips with the huge numbers of people suffering mild to moderate mental health issues, the greater part of the one in four of us affected each year. Applying to this public therapy provision the efficient process design, management and execution more commonly associated with private sector enterprise helped IAPT localities do more for a greater amount of people using their ringfenced investment allocations. Such allocations were substantial; the government provided over £300 million for the first-phase rollout of IAPT in the 2007 spending review.[12]

Psykhe

It was in the pregnant pause between the decision to launch IAPT and the programme's deployment throughout the country that the financial crisis hit. IAPT was rolled out into an economy in recession, but while many public services were required to weather deep cuts, IAPT was largely spared. As expenditure predicated on an expectation of generating far greater savings, IAPT was a policy perfectly attuned to the objectives of austerity. This as much as anything has meant that IAPT has continued to endure for well over a decade, retaining support from administrations of all stripes and outlasting shifting political whims of the sort that had derailed similar initiatives previously. But the programme has not been free of criticism. When IAPT was launched and heralded as a revolutionary initiative, a fact that perhaps escaped due attention was that its target was never to 'meet need', or even get close to doing so. Instead, that Access Target was to establish NHS-commissioned capacity equal to treating just 15 per cent of people who could benefit from therapy. On the face of it, an ambition to treat 15 per cent of the one in four people in need seems unacceptable. Imagine the outcry if it were openly stated that such a small proportion of cancer patients, diabetics, or people presenting at A&E with a broken leg would be funded via the NHS. This is where context matters; one in four of the UK's adult population is roughly 13 million people – an impossible number to reach from a near standing start. Built into the government's own prevalence targets was a tacit acknowledgement of the epidemic scale of the problems faced, and implicit recognition that the perfect could not be allowed to become the enemy of the good in the effort to address them. Given the starting position preceding the IAPT programme it was inevitable that efforts to increase access to therapy would begin somewhere modest, with realistic targets that would not be immediately, catastrophically overwhelmed. Treating 15 per cent of need may have been a compromise ambition, but it was nevertheless a prodigious leap forward. In some localities these fledgling IAPT services, resourced to meet only a fraction of need, quickly attracted criticism over long waiting times, but, like a first morsel of food given to the starving, the fact that the dosage was insufficient did not mean that IAPT was the wrong medicine. With massive pent-up need it was no surprise when the first attempts to sate it failed to touch the sides in some regions. In recent years maturing IAPT services have made great progress bringing waiting times down, and despite a few locality outliers remaining the national programme has brought badly needed ballast to a hitherto patchwork, postcode lottery of provision and waiting times.

After three years, the IAPT programme had reached a million patients and the first major report on its outcomes was produced. After completing therapy, two-thirds of service users had either met the national definition for 'clinical recovery' – their scores reducing below the diagnostic threshold on the questionnaire measures – or had shown at least a statistically significant improvement.[13] Clinically IAPT had proven its effectiveness and, crucially in the interests of the justifying ongoing investment, the early financial results were also positive. More than 45,000 of the first million service users moved off benefits or sick pay and back to work after receiving IAPT treatment.[14] It is impossible to say what would have happened to these people had IAPT never come along, and some would doubtless have regained employment under their own steam. But extrapolating the experience of these first million patients to full-scale rollout, the report estimated savings associated with IAPT of around £272 million a year[15] to the NHS alone, chiefly derived from reduced inpatient bed days, reduction in demand on GPs, and savings in long-term repeat prescriptions for antidepressants.

Twelve years into the programme it is clear that, despite some shortcomings, IAPT has offered meaningful help to immense numbers of people. Help provided free at the point of access that has paid dividends to individuals and to society. In regions where the IAPT framework has manifested the best results, this success has been achieved by pulling off a rare blend of public provision wedded to the best techniques of business, borne along by a conscious culture change that repositioned the concept of 'efficiency' so that it is no longer considered incompatible with care, as was sometimes the case in clinical circles. Historically, psychotherapists have a proud track record of wanting to do their best for patients, arguing that people must get no fewer sessions than they need. This is laudable, but the best IAPT clinicians also extol the importance of giving no *more* sessions than people need. Excessive doses of therapy can build unhelpful dependence, something to avoid in the patient's own interests, and timely discharge also benefits the next person on the waiting list, who is seen more quickly when patient flow is optimised by good productivity. All people are still treated subject to the principle that quality of care remains sacrosanct, but to the fullest extent this condition permits prompt discharge is also valued so that waiting times are minimised and help is provided to people as soon as possible after they have taken the brave step of asking for it. It is with these values uppermost in hearts and minds that IAPT services have made major inroads, helping people with the mild to moderate mental health issues that constitute the great majority of our suggested epidemic.

Integrated IAPT

In 2016 a farsighted second phase of the IAPT programme arrived, geared to overcoming the damaging relics of Cartesian dualism by integrating talking therapies within physical health care settings. 'Integrated IAPT' was an attempt to transcend the narrowly specified structures within which many services operate. The initiative raised the bar for the number of people NHS-commissioned talking therapy services were expected to provide for, increasing it from the aforementioned 15 per cent to 25 per cent. This upscaling included an expectation that some 60 per cent of the marginal layer of new referrals would be made up of people experiencing at least one long-term, comorbid physical health condition – an attempt to address the 'holistic health' issue of intermingled dual dependency between physical and mental health.

In practice, Integrated IAPT has meant transplanting therapists out of their IAPT service hubs and into hospitals, care homes and other specialist settings where people are treated for respiratory, cardiac or musculoskeletal conditions.

Long-term health conditions such as these bring inevitable implications for mental health, and support maintaining a positive mindset can help people struggling with them to better manage their symptoms. By co-locating in this way, real meaning has been given to aspirant buzz words like 'joined-up care'; they become more than just platitudes when people receiving physical health care can leave their treatment room, walk directly into the next, and receive complementary psychological support immediately. Under the Integrated IAPT model work undertaken by a mental health practitioner is reinforced by the active involvement of physical health teams and vice versa, each concerting their efforts to the common aim of holistic care. Integrated IAPT localities are also seeing medical practitioners with different specialisms shadowing each other's clinical sessions to foster a deeper mutual understanding of how their work can be better coordinated, reducing the frequency of frustrating occasions when patients find themselves having to repeat their story over and over to different health workers because they, and their records systems, don't speak directly.

Child and Adolescent Mental Health Services (CAMHS)

The IAPT programme was all about early intervention, the stitch in time that could save nine. The policy helped demonstrate the value of catching people early in the descent into mental ill health and intervening with timely therapy to turn things around. Its good results strengthened the underlying concept that helping individuals in this way helps society at large wherever therapy diverts people away from using the ambulance service, hospitals, the social security system and/or at least six other public utilities still needed to get a tired metaphor about stitches up to the required nine. Once this principle of getting upstream of mental health issues is accepted, and then followed through to its fullest extent, the functioning of our publicly provided Child and Adolescent Mental Health Services (CAMHS) assumes critical importance.

Mental health issues often develop early, and in the UK one in every nine children aged five to fifteen is reckoned to have a mental health disorder.[16] Half of all mental health problems are established by age fourteen, and three-quarters by twenty-four.[17] Suicide rates among the UK's children and young people are now bucking the general trend that has seen numbers falling among the whole population since 2000. Data released by the Office of National Statistics in 2018 showed that suicide rates among girls and young women aged fifteen to nineteen have climbed to their highest levels since reliable records began in 1981. Suicide rates among males of the same age are also rising, despite suicides among men of older ages declining steadily.[18] In this context children's mental health services must be an investment priority, as the source of the earliest opportunities to make those vital, life-changing interventions for individuals – and the biggest savings for the Exchequer. But their bean counters must have missed the memo on the financial case for this one, as the UK's children's mental health services find themselves in a worse state of underinvestment than their adult equivalents.

Shortly after IAPT had been rolled out, an NHS initiative to mirror it with a counterpart programme for children and young people was attempted. 'Young People's

IAPT' had the same evidence-based principles and lofty aspirations as its parent template, but not the same level of ringfenced funding dedicated to training a new workforce of children's specialists to uplift capacity at scale. In the absence of requisite funding, CAMHS services did their best to shift their practices towards the IAPT model, but no real movement was achieved, more the reflex jerking usually associated with a well-placed spoon to the knee. Children's services, already overloaded, found themselves with extra expectations but no more resources to meet them, and the initiative was allowed to wither quietly with all air sucked out of it. Today, underfunded CAMHS services have been left little option but to respond by pulling up the drawbridge, setting prohibitively high access criteria as a means of dealing with overwhelming demand and waiting lists that they simply are not equipped to handle. Theirs is a vital job, but if we don't give them the tools they cannot be expected to do it. According to a 2018 report by the Association of Child Psychotherapists, the state of CAMHS now amounts to a 'silent catastrophe',[19] a 'serious and worsening crisis' resulting from prolonged underfunding that has brought growing risks of inappropriate reliance on emergency departments, and ultimately even of suicides resulting from the inaccessibility of care.

Crisis Care

Another component of the mental health care system often singled out for all the wrong reasons is crisis provision – care for people who are seriously mentally unwell, who may present a high risk of harming themselves or others, and who cannot be adequately treated on an outpatient basis. In England the number of NHS mental health inpatient beds has been falling for decades, reducing from 68,000 in 1988 to just 18,400 in 2019.[20] This trend is of course influenced by its proximity to the latter phases of deinstitutionalisation, when people were brought out of asylums and into the community. But an evolving model of care has not been the only factor behind falling bed numbers; inpatient services remain the most expensive element of the mental health care landscape, and budget cuts have also been driving the trend. Beds cannot be cut indefinitely; even with a well-functioning, community-based model a minimum level of inpatient architecture must be maintained to cater for the most serious, urgent cases that inevitably arise. At present capacity, bed shortages frequently force NHS trusts to send patients away from their home regions to beds elsewhere – so-called out-of-area placements. Sometimes trusts are forced to search hundreds of miles for an available bed, and this can bring damaging consequences. When people who are seriously ill are relocated in the midst of crisis, far away from whatever family and support networks may otherwise have offered stability and comfort, their distress can be exacerbated and their recovery prospects impaired. Out-of-area placements can carry damaging economic implications too; if no suitable NHS bed is found, trusts sometimes have no option but to pay supernormal profits to private providers who are able to supply one. In these circumstances, cuts to NHS services that would otherwise have done the job at far lower cost are shown up as clumsy policy and false economy.

In combination with the gross overstretch faced by children's services, this condition of crisis care makes for a damning picture of the UK's mental health system. Until these things are fixed, 'parity of esteem' will remain a pipedream. We *should* esteem the importance of mental health as highly as physical health because, as the national strategy frames it, there is 'no health without mental health'. For that very reason, parity of investment is now just as important as parity of esteem.

United States Policy

In the United States the picture is even more complex, and, for individuals in need, access to therapy even less certain. In 1955 Congress passed the Mental Health Study Act, leading to the establishment of the Joint Commission on Mental Illness and Mental Health. Its 1961 report 'Action for Mental Health' anticipated a transformed landscape of deinstitutionalised, community-based care, accompanied by a publicly funded programme to raise awareness of mental health issues. President Kennedy's subsequent 'New Frontier' package of social and economic reforms then included an attempt to deliver this community integration. Signed into law in 1963, the Community Mental Health Act provided state grants to be used establishing a network of local mental health centres that would replace the asylums, ushering in a system where patients could be treated while living in their own homes and participating in society. But the division of federal and state responsibilities created an extra disconnect that diluted the original vision of the legislation, as responsibility for delivering it was devolved to the states. Not all of the proposed centres were built, and many that were built went underfunded – some states taking the opportunity to relieve stretched budgets by closing expensive hospitals and retaining the savings instead of spending proportionately on community care. Then, in the aftermath of the economic crash, states have cut a further $4 billion in public mental health funding collectively since 2008.[21]

Under the present insurance-based healthcare model, millions of Americans are now denied access to mental health care through lack of means to pay for it. The obligations created by deinstitutionalisation have not been met, and prisons and nursing homes have become default warehouses for those in psychological distress, packed with people washed down the overflow pipe of a blocked mental health system. Attempts to dispel mental health stigma have also been more heated in the United States, where the issue of mental health has been raised repeatedly in the course of wrestling with national angst over gun crime. Is it really the guns that are the problem? Or is it the people wielding them, who are just mentally ill? The political debate has often fallen short of due balance, misrepresenting people as mentally ill, and the mentally ill as inevitably dangerous, generating more heat than light. This is one among a small number of blemishes that has disrupted the pattern of slow but otherwise steady progress in Western societies towards a culture of greater mental health awareness, one that finally overcomes the inveterate habit of stigmatising sufferers as 'the other' – the witless, the feckless and the hapless, people to be scorned, feared or shamed.

Stigma

Anonymity in good works may be a high-order virtue, but it doesn't wash when it comes to mental health. Talking about mental health issues helps, and knowing help is available also helps. So combatting stigma is important too; it lets people know that mental ill health is not abnormal, and is no cause for shame. In moments of dark despair it takes great courage to find the strength to ask for help. When people are struggling to gather that courage it is vital they feel able to seek help without fear of judgement or censure, whether from family, friends or anyone else. Unless they feel secure in this they may not ask *at all*, and so become victims of the stigma impediment. Overcoming this stigma is important, because the difference between someone feeling able to reach out or not is sometimes the difference between a life saved or a life lost. This is why the messages we consume about mental health from the media have always mattered, whether from social media now or from the texts of Shakespeare generations ago. Popular culture has always steered ambient attitudes. The stigma impediment is also why it is so damaging when people rush to judge, misrepresenting mental ill health as a weakness, or some personal or moral failing, rather than what it really is – something that can affect anyone. Every occasion on which someone speaks of mental ill health in pejorative terms is another little blow chipping away at the precious, fragile edifice that is our collective security in our own skins.

Men especially now face a particular issue with stigma. In every one of the thirty-five regions I had the privilege of serving as a provider of NHS-commissioned therapy services the numbers confirmed that story with uncanny consistency. Among the thousands of people passing through the doors of these services each month, receiving psychological therapies from our teams, the picture was the same – when patient demographics were analysed, two-thirds of service users were routinely female, and only a third male. Whether in Canterbury, Newcastle, Liverpool, Peterborough, Nottingham or any other corner of the country the split remained a near constant. Consistently a two-to-one gender ratio repeated, with no locality departing from the rule by more than a handful of percentage points, and barely a scintilla of dissonance when the figures were tracked over time. At first this unerring symmetry surprised – could women really be more predisposed to mental ill health than men? Then I came to realise that I was witnessing the stigma impediment, made visible through the law of large numbers. Men have no special resistance to mental ill health; they are simply less likely to come forward.

Sadly the effects of stigma are also visible in official suicide statistics. Data from the Office for National Statistics shows that men in most age brackets are approximately 50 per cent more likely to die by their own hand than women,[22] and the numbers are rising. In England, 3,800 deaths were registered as suicide among men of all ages in 2018, up from 3,328 in 2017.[23] Stigma can affect people from all demographics and any social stratum, but women have done a better job of overcoming it to face up to their feelings. Men, in contrast, remain particularly sensitive to stigma and disproportionately reluctant to access treatment for mental health issues as a result, concerned that admitting an issue might somehow invalidate their manhood in the eyes of their peers. While some have now come around to considering the naked truth a good thing, many still see only indecency. There remains a macho rhythm to the resting pulse of masculinity that is causing men to repress emotions, to feel that any vulnerability must be hidden, and it is allowing conversations to go unspoken. Our culture needs to find a way to overcome this, so that men feel able to let go of these inhibitions, and free to seek help when they need it.

Despite this, the struggle against the negative stigma that has historically attached to mental health is one sphere where steady progress has been made. The publicity generated by World Mental Health Day, now going for more than a quarter of a century, has been a contributing factor, and the message has steadily snowballed. Mental health is now a subject that attracts column inches the year round, with an ever growing army of public figures rallying to the cause. But perhaps most powerful have been the shared accounts, celebrity or not, of personal struggles with mental health. These personal testimonies have the power to embolden and inspire others who are navigating desperate times of their own. And as mental ill health has stepped out from behind the veil to become a more normalised topic of conversation, the once commonplace occasions when the language of mental health was casually repurposed and employed pejoratively in schools and workplaces are also, thankfully, diminishing. Ironically, this progress may be another factor fuelling perceptions that we are suffering a modern epidemic of mental ill health, as problems that were always present but once hidden have shed taboo status and emerged into the light of our collective awareness. Ultimately this is a good thing, and the difference it has made to people suffering, and to those working in health services trying to help them, feels almost tangible. In the early 2000s telling someone you worked in mental health might have provoked a raised eyebrow, a subtle and unspoken 'Why would you?' Today there is widespread acceptance that mental health matters, a broad recognition that good mental health is a fundamental prerequisite for a good life and a necessary platform for the outcomes other enterprises like our housing and education services, or the criminal justice system are striving to achieve. Mental health has become no less than the front line where the good fight for human well-being is fought.

11

O BRAVE NEW WORLD! – A FUTURE

Since earliest civilisation, mental ill health has alarmed, fascinated and confounded humanity. We have groped in darkness to understand and treat illnesses that are largely invisible, and though scientific breakthroughs have improved our knowledge of the brain, and advances in treatment have eased psychological distress for many, there is much we still don't understand, and even more that we have yet to master. Innumerable questions still remain – about causation, the interplay of biopsychosocial factors, and why treatments that work for some do not satisfy others. It will likely be ages before all questions are answered, all secrets revealed, and our knowledge of the mind's operations clicks into place to be fully understood – if full understanding is even attainable.

A Modern Epidemic?

Are we, in the here and now, experiencing a modern epidemic of mental ill health? With huge gaps in the evidence base, room for speculation will remain and any simple answer must be controversial and unsatisfactory. But so is sitting on the fence. On balance, then, let us acknowledge that we *are* suffering a modern epidemic of mental ill health, but also acknowledge that it cannot be proven that this epidemic is exclusively modern. In fact, it probably isn't – this particular manifestation of the pale horse has likely always stalked humanity, may even be an intrinsic part of what it is to *be* human, and the proportion of us suffering with mental ill health now may well be similar to what it has always been.

Trying to get hold of mental health is like trying to grasp the proverbial greased piglet, but it can help to visualise mental health as a spectrum with the unicorn of perfect health coupled with perfect bliss at one pole, the majority of people coping near the middle, and a graduated range of 'threshold met' diagnosable mental illnesses at the other extreme. We are all, in fact, on a continuous motion back and forth along this spectrum throughout our lives. Our individual bandwidths differ, and sometimes major life events might come along to pitch us beyond our usual parameters; occasionally we may even tip across the threshold beyond which a professional might decide that we could benefit from help. Some people may be more prone to this tipping over than others, having a greater mental health elasticity, to appropriate a term from the economist's toolbox, indicating a higher propensity and underlying vulnerability to mental ill health.

Imagining all our individual patterns overlaid in aggregate along this spectrum provides a heat map of the human condition that helps overcome the ephemeral nature of community mental health. If the 'diagnosability' line at the extreme of this collective picture is set too narrowly it sucks everything but the most tepid behaviour into a diagnosis of illness. Making the opposite error, not drawing a line at all, may seem inclusive but sets us down the path already trodden by anti-psychiatry, with the same risk that help is denied to those with underestimated needs. This is where the moveable feast of context leaves proof of our epidemic hypothesis holed beneath the waterline – thresholds have shifted over time, tracking fluid perceptions of what counts as abnormal behaviour and an evolving definition of what mental illness entails. Cultural anthropology is sufficiently woolly that attempting to prove the case that mental ill health has risen down the centuries is to pile 'ifs' on top of 'buts'. But irrespective of whether incidence of mental ill health is now on the upslope beyond a historic resting rate, or the downslope away from it, what we do know is that one in four people will experience some form of psychological ill health this year, and one in six are doing so right now. These numbers certainly do constitute an epidemic in the here and now, and the sufferers deserve help today. This is the dominating fact, and our spur to action.

Beyond this top-level conclusion it is still possible to pinpoint some simple but useful truths capable of being translated into practical action and policy. We know that some mental ill health conditions are undoubtedly more nature than nurture, a natural prevalence inherent to humanity that will likely always be around. But we also know that some mental ill health, particularly mild to moderate issues, can take hold in response to the onslaught of events, the ups and downs of life's rich tapestry as we each weave our own little patterns through this shared experience we call life. Bio-psycho-social factors all impact our mental health, and all have the potential to pitch our markers closer to the extremes of our spectrum, for better or for worse. Taking the long view, we may not be able to prove whether mental ill health is trending positively or negatively, but the kaleidoscopic forces acting upon our collective mental health today are undeniably unprecedented.

So what are the factors making today's world different? Four major socioeconomic forces have coincided, creating a uniquely modern combination: globalisation hitting the buffers in the wake of an economic crash; the ascent of our digital lives, where the air seems to be getting thinner and thinner; less well-balanced lifestyles and diets; and the attrition of religious beliefs that once acted as a glue, helping hold life together for generations past. A compounding factor has been the *allegrissimo* urgency with which these transfigurative forces have combined. Technological advancement in particular has been exponential, and today *the great world spins forever down the ringing grooves of change*[1] at a tempo never previously known. It is a pace that may simply be outstripping the capacity of many to adapt, and we are now buckling under the growing pains of this over-rapid change. These modern forces may not have moved the underlying organic rate of people suffering the most severe and enduring forms of mental ill health, but they are the triggers now driving the patterns flying about the mid-zones of our mind's-eye spectrum, exerting influence on the rate of the moderate mental health issues that constitute the great bulk of the one-in-four statistic, just as the environments inhabited by our ancestors would have influenced prevalence in their times.

At the macro level, attempting to weigh each factor to pin blame on any one above others is like trying to pin jelly to the wall. The combination is key. Academic institutions teach biology, psychology, economics, sociology, religious studies and the technologies as separate subjects, but out in the real world these disciplines mix together to shape the human experience. The act of mixing is not like placing marbles in a jar, shaking it, and watching each orbit the other; it is like pouring differently coloured paints into the jar and seeing them blend to a new shade. The precise tone created is a signature unique to our age; it is the blend colouring mental health in our society today, and once the paints are mixed no element can easily be reversed out, isolated again and cleanly plucked from the jar as a marble might be. In the modern mix, every component discipline is undergoing rapid change, so the blend is morphing quickly too; and because this combination is now mutating with uniquely ultra-modern pace, a growing mismatch has developed between the complex biopsychosocial forces affecting our societies and the slower to adapt architecture of the social and political institutions intended to sustain us within them. Our health and social care systems and the extant corpus of legislation that underpins them are now straining to manage new-world problems against the grain of old-world structures that are still geared towards material world problems, not digital dimensions, and working in silos, not collaborating beyond boundaries. In our connected world, global economic woes, inequality, climate change and the Covid-19 pandemic are now supranational problems, beyond the control of any individual nation state; little wonder governments are struggling and their populations feeling the strain. But the extant international system of political and economic institutions also appears toothless in the face of these problems, and no one yet knows how to begin protecting human wellbeing in the cloud, where national borders mean nothing and a lie can travel all the way around the world, perhaps several times, while the truth is still lacing its boots.[2]

The Future

The struggle to understand mental health is intertwined with the eternal struggle to understand human nature. The reality is that we remain quite near the start of this struggle, and early on in the journey towards learning how to build lives and lifestyles that give the best chance of optimising mental health for all. When Hippocrates was winning Greek hearts and minds towards the idea of natural, rather than supernatural causes for mental ill health, he was doing so some 6,000 years after the dates of the earliest known trepanation patients. We think of Hippocrates as a giant of the ancient world, but in the vast ocean of time his wave broke far more closely to ours than it did theirs. With this perspective, and while still striving to improve mental health, we should accept too that it is a struggle that will remain part of humanity's story for a long time to come. Perhaps the struggle *is* the story – the spectre of human frailty ever at our backs, as indivisible from ourselves as our very DNA. If so, we must learn to manage our mental health and to live with it. We certainly won't live without it. If we ever did learn to eradicate psychological distress, perhaps we would also have learned not to be human. Time for Sisyphus to stop rolling his boulder up the hill.

A morsel of comfort follows from the thought that the present spotlight on mental health is an indication that Western society has reached a point where basic needs for food, safety and survival are, for most, routinely met to such a degree that good mental health is now given increasing prominence in societies that care enough to value it. But if we could sponge clear the vista and start again, what could be done to improve the odds of well-being? What does it even mean to 'live well' as a human being in the twenty-first century? A good starting point might be to consider how an updated hierarchy of needs might look if Maslow was composing one today. Our nucleus of needs remains the same; we are still dependent on shelter, safety and sustenance, and still living in societies where not everyone can rely on them. But more people than ever before *can*, and so are concerned with the hierarchy's upper reaches as a result. These upper reaches are where the socioeconomic conditions for self-fulfilment are changing the fastest.

With consumerism now globalised, digitised and beating its massive chest, the starting point in the journey to fulfilment feels further back to people for whom material metrics are the mainspring of satisfaction. There is so much to aspire to, and such heightened awareness of it all. Technology that would have seemed godlike to our ancestors has not – yet, at least – delivered the high-end contentment Maslow described, and has not solved the problems of human well-being. Instead it has supersized them in a new dimension and afforded billions a glimpse of the 'just maybe', and maybe that is really the root of what is going on. Certainly the early twenty-first century feels like one of history's crossroads. *Brave New World* was the title of Aldous Huxley's dystopian novel of 1931, a vision of the future that imagined a world state, technologically enforced coercive control, happiness derived from pills, and a subclass of 'savages' abandoned to live outside the new world order. This fiction will feel eerily portentous for many today, but it is not the only possible blueprint for humanity's future, and it is not too late to turn things around. Shakespeare's original vision from *The Tempest* offers more optimism for human potential:

> O wonder!
> How many goodly creatures are there here,
> How beauteous mankind is!
> O brave new world, that has such people in it.[3]

While we cannot expect to eradicate mental ill health, one important implication of the biopsychosocial understanding of the modern epidemic, and of our mind's-eye spectrum, is that the factors contributing to it *are* susceptible to manipulation. We can hope to minimise mental ill health in future by the choices we make next, both individually and collectively. Policy offers the possibility of nudging society towards the right or the wrong extremity, something underappreciated as the trammelled lines of Cartesian dualism were ploughed and re-ploughed through centuries in which holistic health was largely overlooked. By developing fresh support structures appropriate to modern life, it should be possible to retune our living conditions to be more compatible with good mental health: a fresh blend of technology, responsibility, ingenuity and compassion that leaves fewer people excluded. We are richer than ever before and enjoy greater opportunities and life expectancy than ever before. We should not denounce the systems that got us here - that ideological struggle was lost with the Luddites - but two centuries on from those industrial revolution saboteurs we could be doing more to manage the human fallout of the new digital revolution and full-throttle globalised capitalism. When Henry Ford rolled out his Model T, the history of automobile development didn't stop there; we got traffic laws, safety belts, air bags, speed limits and eventually catalytic converters and electric cars to better align new technology and the common good. Without this vigilant spirit of continuous improvement, the 'on the shoulders of giants' nature of technological advancement will occasionally lead to unintended risks, and to unacceptable consequences. Today, we must be careful not to thoughtlessly arrange ourselves into a circular firing squad.

Once the potential for the majority towards the middle of society's mental health spectrum to shift is acknowledged, it begs the question of how we should measure the extent to which the societies we have built, or arrived at, in that semi organic process beyond the compass of any individual agent, are well matched with well-being. When gauging how their citizens are faring, post-war politicians have routinely turned to economic metrics, particularly gross domestic product (GDP), as their standard. GDP is the market value of the total output produced by an economy each year. For economists, and for politicians assuming offices of state, GDP appears so early in their learning curve that it goes unquestioned, a building block so fundamental it has become part of the political furniture. But the pre-eminence afforded to GDP in questions of policy relies on a fundamental assumption that when the economy is doing well the country is doing well too, and so are the people living within it. While this may hold in broad terms, GDP is a coarse-grained measure. It reveals national wealth in totality, but illuminates nothing about its distribution, about health, happiness or anything whatsoever not financially oriented that might still matter to people going about their lives. Monomania over GDP also offers no safeguards against hidden, increasingly problematic externality costs, environmental degradation included.

Perhaps we should aspire to a new measure, one that transcends models of markets to model human experience. The objective would not be to replace GDP or other monetary metrics but to create a companion measure to moderate the financial ones. The complementary measure could be an index of human well-being, to inform the recalibration needed to keep the neoliberal economic model fit for modern challenges. Constituent parts of this well-being measure could include health outcomes; a physical activity index; a count of opportunities to socialise, access green space and breathe pollution-free air; and perhaps sampled, self-reported well-being scales as adopted by the IAPT programme. The World Health Organisation's WHO-5 mental well-being index, comprising five questions about feeling cheerful, calm, active, rested and interested, could be adopted as another component, bringing the possibility of facilitating international comparison. To account for the thread running between poverty and mental health some financial components could also be included within this holistic measure, with factors like of child poverty and income inequality attributed a value to be weighed in the balance alongside the other constituent parts. Would things improve if future chancellors had not one but two first-order measures to report on? National GDP *pari passu* with national well-being? Such a system would certainly create fresh checks and balances to the financial yardstick of progress. At the moment we have the yin without the yang, and a fraying social fabric as perceptions of injustice and inequality fester.

Financial prudence must remain. Incentivising the productivity that generates wealth will always be essential and profit is not a bad thing, especially when surplus is put to a just purpose. The incentives to productive enterprise may actually become *greater* in circumstances where everyone can transparently see the wellbeing, as well as the financial, dividends of a strong economy accruing back to them. We should care about prosperity, but we should also care about how the fruits of it are spent, elevating human well-being in the minds of policymakers and providing a tool for attuning society more harmoniously with it. In the long term, the thinking need not be limited to valuing only human well-being but could be extended so its units are weighted to include all life, finding synergy with efforts already underway to halt species extinction and limit carbon emissions before the consequences are irreversible.

Achieving all this would require major cultural change, but opportunities exist for iteratively guiding the course of our well-being and mental health for the better. We must aim for the 'natural rate' where mental ill health is minimised as much as possible, with the question 'what will this do to well-being?' asked by standing convention whenever major issues are debated in the corridors of power. We need a society of caring capitalism, where the benefits of our modern genius are more evenly shared, and where fewer are left behind. This may sound like a castle in the air, but New Zealand has already become the first country to put well-being, not growth or production, at the centre of its economic policy. Prime Minister Jacinda Ardern set out details of a prototype 'Well-being Budget' for New Zealand at the 2019 World Economics Forum in Davos, specifying 'thriving in the digital age; improving mental health services; reducing child poverty; developing a low-emission, sustainable economy; and addressing inequality'[4] as five domains by which success would be measured. Whether this bold move is ultimately judged a seminal example for others to follow or a failed experiment remains to be seen, but calls for 'purposeful capitalism' are strengthening elsewhere, including in the United States, Europe and the United Arab Emirates, which now even boasts a Minister of State for Happiness. To avoid being tokenistic, such initiatives require clear scope and substantial powers. Real, sustained change will require even more, no less than an existential transformation to re-orientate our whole political DNA, and one achieved without impairing economic productivity or creating burdens on free markets – the engine that must pay for it.

Policy

Preventing mental ill health by recalibrating societies to better promote positive mental health is the panacea objective. Irons are in the fire, and some are getting warm, but reconditioning society takes time; overhauling the bedrock principles of a dominant economic philosophy is no easy process. While the heavy lifting is being done there are more immediate, practical actions that can still be taken within the constraints of existing infrastructure – by politicians, by corporations and by each of us as individuals. Governments have a uniquely privileged opportunity, and parallel responsibility, to use their legislative powers to help people who find themselves in distress right now. We must continue along the development curve of recent decades, pursuing the objective of providing appropriate, dignified and compassionate community care services for people whose lives have been blighted by mental health conditions. There is no easy or inexpensive shortcut for this – it requires public investment, and warrants it too. So the amplification of the UK's IAPT programme, and especially support for its lateral diversification into co-location with physical health, must continue. It makes no sense to change horses when the evidence is clear that the policy is working. Children and young people's mental health is now the arena where fresh initiatives, greater investment and the livelier attention of government is most urgently required. The long waiting lists and high treatment thresholds that have bedevilled children's services must be cut away, and services reformed with a root-and-branch reshaping. This will require new pathways, predicated on the rapid-response mentality that minimises waiting time.

The main determinant of an individual's propensity to respond to therapy is the waiting time they experience from referral to assessment, then assessment to treatment. In 2013, asked to help clear a waiting list of a thousand people who had been waiting a year for NHS therapy on the south coast, our charity made arrangements to bring capacity to the area, then telephoned and contacted everyone on the list seeking to book them in for an appointment. A year on from their original referral, most didn't respond at all either to calls or letters, and were referred back to their GP, and only 10 per cent ended up receiving therapy. The equivalent statistic can reach as high as 90 per cent in well-grooved services where the waiting time from referral to therapy is measured in days, not years, so that people get timely help when they need it. If there are no waiting lists then people won't give up hope of ever receiving help and vote with their feet. Nor can they get worse while on a waiting list, adding pressure to other parts of the public system. Most importantly, they can't die on a waiting list either, as tragically sometimes happens when people facing long queues for therapy take their own lives.

To overcome these challenges, young people's mental health services require vastly greater investment. Even in straitened times, when it may not be possible to satisfy all claims, we can at least cover the vital bases and eat our lumps elsewhere. Children's mental health is a vital base, and expenditure here doesn't just help us today – tomorrow's taxpayers benefit too. Upskilling teachers, arming them with greater understanding and resources, would also aid the effort to improve young people's mental health. Teachers do not need retraining as therapists, just equipping with enough understanding of 'mental health first aid' to recognise signs of burgeoning mental health issues, and to respond when they do encounter them – even if the response is as simple as facilitating a speedy referral into a service that is equipped to offer help. Young people themselves should also be taught the knowledge and skills to look after their own mental health. While progress has been made with this, it remains an aspiration when it should be a universal minimum, and educational establishments offer an ideal forum where young people could be better engaged.

Another chance of a quick win is in the creation of a national, twenty-four-seven NHS helpline for people of any age struggling with mental ill health. The Samaritans occupy similar turf and offer valuable support, but in the absence of common IT systems they remain semi-detached from the NHS services that provide the longer-term therapy many of their callers really need, and ultimately go on to receive. The Samaritans' work ought to be augmenting national helpline capacity, not relied upon as the mainstay of it. A publicly commissioned equivalent, operating on the same patient records systems as the NHS, would facilitate warm transfers directly into NHS therapy appointments on a live call. Available round-the-clock, such a service could stem the flow into emergency departments of people whose issues are primarily psychological, but who have nowhere else to turn. This is not to disparage the principle of non-NHS organisations providing health services; all available talent and capacity should be harnessed. However, talk of opening up the NHS often raises disquiet. The suggestion that United States corporations have eyes on the NHS, eager to feast on the dripping roast of our public healthcare services, generates particular agitation among those concerned that privatisation will rip the soul from them. In truth, privatisation has been underway for years. In recent decades dozens of NHS psychological therapy services have been offered up for open tender by NHS commissioners. Any organisation, public, private or charitable, is free to bid for these services on a basis of fair and transparent competition. Ours did, and thirty-five NHS commissioning localities chose us as their provider, almost all of the resulting contracts having been previously delivered directly by one NHS trust or other. As a charitable provider, any profit we made was reinvested into front-line services – surplus for a purpose. And free of stultifying public sector overheads, the services could be delivered in a more cost-effective way, delivering more good for more people from the same fixed investment, and without dilution of quality.

But despite examples of successful collaboration between the NHS and independent providers, privatisation of care remains anathema to many who point to examples where it has gone badly wrong, as with the allegations of neglect and abuse that emerged in the course of a BBC investigation into the Castlebeck scandal of 2011.[5] Saddening though such cases are, historical problems with privatisation have not rested in the concept but the execution. The NHS is a national institution to be cherished and a core of NHS services should always be preserved. But a mixed economy of provision, where voluntary organisations in particular are welcomed into the fold to bring their own skills, specialisms and capacity, offers the best of all worlds, helping health systems to tap into an extended talent pool and to integrate more closely with the communities they serve, ultimately to the benefit of the public. A mixed provider landscape involves interfaces, and so some risk of patients falling between services, but no more so than if separate NHS organisations were left delivering them. Common IT systems and information-sharing protocols are the real trick to overcoming this, and such an approach is long overdue. Harnessing 'all the talents' in this way, without haemorrhaging profits through the nose to private providers, is a task that is well within the ken of NHS commissioners. Already many NHS-commissioned psychological therapy services are remunerated on a per case basis, according to clinical sessions delivered and with going rates of just a few hundred pounds per case – rates that barely allow room for therapists' salaries, let alone cream skimming by shareholders up the chain.

Opportunities clearly exist to improve the current mental health care system. But beyond policies like these we cannot rely solely on legislators to deliver the changes needed in a world evolving too fast for sclerotic legislation to keep pace. Transient governments, thinking in majorities as the baton of power passes from one administration to the next, are outmatched by the forces gushing over them. Achieving a well-being rebalance that permeates universally, and becomes baked in, will oblige every participant in our society to rise to the task. This means governments and public institutions, but it also means every business, every employer, and each of us as individuals.

Corporations

Large social media providers are magnates of the modern age. Their success has placed vast wealth and resources at their command. Should they have an obligation to harness these resources to promote their customers' well-being? The potential is enormous, and goes beyond reactive policing to moderate illegal or negative content on their platforms. If ambitions were raised, these platforms could utilise their wealth of data to proactively pursue positive ends. If click habits and content choices enable them to identify which products to push on us, maybe the algorithms behind this could be adapted to gauge whether someone is at a low ebb, at risk, or in need of support. Information could then be displayed about the options for getting appropriate help, whether with addiction problems, relationship issues, mental health concerns or anything else. A safe, facilitated space could be offered where like-minded platform users, wrestling with similar issues, could connect to benefit from peer support in a moderated, therapeutic environment. If the inherent rightness of social media providers using their immense reach to promote positive mental health isn't sufficient incentive of itself, the possibility offers an obvious PR opportunity at a time when platforms are under scrutiny over dubious data harvesting and safeguarding practices. In the competition for clicks there would surely be rewards for those that participate responsibly, harnessing their technologies for altruistic ends and treating their customers as more than counted consumption beans.

Corporations should have even greater interest in promoting the well-being of their own staff. Particular sensitivities and stigma can accompany mental health issues in workplaces. In pressured circumstances it is natural that we will at times feel stressed, anxious or depressed, and it is in everybody's interest that this is addressed – most profoundly so that help can be made available to individuals in times of need. But employers too are better served by a healthy, productive workforce than one characterised by anxiety, stress and low levels of well-being. Unresolved mental health issues cause sickness absence, reduced productivity and high staff turnover, and employers bear the associated costs – paying someone else to cover a staff member on long-term sick leave, or advertising to replace someone who has become overwhelmed and quit. Making well-being services – confidential helplines, counselling and critical incident support – available to staff helps avoid this by intervening before issues spiral to crisis point. Employers offering these benefits enjoy a competitive advantage, particularly in recruitment and retention. There are, of course, plenty of beneficent employers around already, and workplace innovations like access to subsidised private healthcare and flexible working hours have already enhanced work-life balance for millions. As the digitally driven second age of capitalism matures, the time is now ripe for all employers – big business especially – to push the frontiers even further, welcoming a more ethical settlement for all those units of consumption and production they depend upon, so that everyone is treated with compassion and as a whole person, with all the needs and vulnerabilities real people have.

Compassion

Now is also a good place in our journey to consider a rebalance for our own personal well-being, and that of others. These personal recalibrations will need to involve finding peace with our social media consumption, and the impact of the digital revolution on our work-life balance. The internet is an extraordinarily powerful yet fiendishly addictive new toy, and those of us who have overused it since it burst into being must find a way to step back from the precipice, regulating consumption to find a more comfortable relationship that preserves the upsides while safeguarding against obsession and addiction. If we don't like being bombarded with bad news stories, maybe we should click the good ones instead. If digital life becomes overwhelming, perhaps we should try disconnecting. And if part of the problem is that we are really hunter-gatherer imposters pursuing sedentary routines in conflict with our animalistic biology, perhaps simply getting out of doors more is part of the answer too.

Finally, there is the simple truth that If we don't like how society views and treats mental health, we each have the power to start changing it. Society's prevailing attitude is only the aggregate of all our individual thoughts and deeds. If it needs improving, then solving this part of the conundrum is within our collective control. We can all help by carrying our values on our tongues, by challenging pejorative attitudes to mental health whenever we encounter them, by remembering and including neighbours, friends or relatives who may be lonely or depressed and by easing the burden of each other's many modern pressures with greater consideration and understanding in the workplace and at home. None of us are required to give a moment's thought to the well-being of a stranger – but is it too much to ask? The moment we let go of our own fears and take a leap of altruistic trust may be the moment a corner is turned. Little day-to-day kindnesses are important; they can have the power to change lives, even to save them. The struggle for mental health may remain a fitful, circuitous journey for eons to come, but we can take inspiration from the knowledge that we are all of us together capable of turning the tide in this struggle, through the simple power of compassion.

HOPE – AN EPILOGUE

Through 1665 and the infamous year of 1666, the Pale Horse's most notorious foot soldier was at large. In London the spread was rampant, but elsewhere England's rural communities remained mostly untouched, and for people in the small Derbyshire village of Eyam life passed serenely unblemished – until a visitor visited a blemish on that serenity. The Plague's containment all changed when a merchant brought it north from the capital and into Eyam, carried by fleas hidden in a consignment of cloths. When its first victim developed the tell-tale swellings, then died the agonising death of plague, the terrible realisation that Black Death had arrived in isolated Eyam must have hit its residents like a hammer blow. Their first instinct was to run, to get out as quickly as possible, and save themselves from any more risk of infection. Instead, inspired by local rector William Mompesson, they chose another way. Once the initial panic had abated, the thought rising uppermost in local minds was that theirs was an isolated settlement of hundreds, surrounded by much larger towns of many thousands – places that would become defenceless breeding grounds for the Plague should it be allowed to spread. So, the people of Eyam chose to cordon themselves off in quarantine, deciding collectively that no one should come or go from the village until the threat had passed.

The punishment the Plague exacted for this defiance was savage. Eyam's population was ravaged. Two hundred and sixty had died before the Plague was done,[1] more than half Eyam's original population by some estimates. No one, not even the few survivors, had been left untouched. They had endured appalling losses. Elizabeth Hancock, for instance, had been forced to drag the bodies of her husband and six young children, one after another in the space of just eight days, into a neighbouring field where she buried them herself, having no alternative in her grim isolation. For families like hers, the temptation to flee this village of the damned, as Eyam quickly became known, must have been tremendous. But in spite of the most extreme hardships and loss, the will of Eyam's people would not break. Their legacy would be glorious. The monumental sacrifices of these hundreds succeeded in preventing the Plague reaching the many, many thousands living in the larger settlements of Derbyshire and Yorkshire on their doorstep. Eyam is one of history's most powerful examples of human suffering and endurance. And in their adversity the people there also gave us one of the greatest demonstrations of humanity itself – offering up their own lives so that others, strangers to them, would be spared.

We all face adversity in life. The coming of Covid-19 has recently given the world a reminder of the sort of perils that periodically beset our ancestors. With the virus and its financial fallout looking set to blight communities for some time yet to come, the scale of mental ill health in those communities has been amplified yet further, and the nature of it altered yet again. New health anxieties, new financial anxieties and new bereavements are creating a whole new lived reality for modern populations to navigate, reminding us all of just how precious and just how fragile our existence really is.

At whatever level you encounter adversity, don't give up. There may be times when we feel things are too much, and *want to*, but never, never, never give up. Better is always possible. As children we think the dramas of youth mean everything, until we grow up and realise they didn't. As adults we think we know who we are, for better or worse, until our innermost selves surprise us, and we realise we don't. A compass always points due north, until once every 200,000 to 300,000 years the poles reverse, and suddenly it doesn't. The swim against the tide has long been the grist to humanity's mill. In the twenty-first century we have fought our way to technological genius that has earned us the freedoms of gods, and we must now choose whether to use it to liberate us or shut ourselves in. When you are at your lowest ebb, lend help to someone in greater need. When you feel weak, remember that weaknesses lose their edge once we let go of our own concerns, and replace them with concern for others. Time is precious. So is health. So is life, in every breath. These are constants that won't shift. Human nature can be magnificent.

FIGURES

Fig. 1. Official Suicide Rates in the UK 1982 to 2018 (Deaths per 100,000 Persons*)

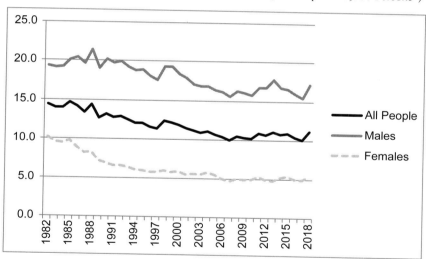

*Using the National ONS definition of suicide. Age standardised suicide rates per 100,000 is the ONS measure; standardised to the European Standard Population 2013. According to the ONS Age-standardised rates are used to *'allow comparison between populations that may contain different proportions of people of different ages'*.

Source: Office for National Statistics, Suicides in the UK: 2018 registrations: Registered deaths in the UK from suicide analysed by sex, age, area of usual residence of the deceased and suicide method, published 2019.

Fig. 2. United States Suicide Rates 2008 to 2017 (Deaths per 100,000 Persons)

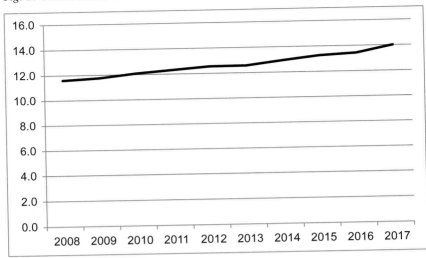

Source: American Foundation for Suicide Prevention, 'Suicide Statistics' Web Resource.

Fig. 3. UK Suicides per 100,000 Population in 2018 by Age Range and Gender, Including among Children and Young People*

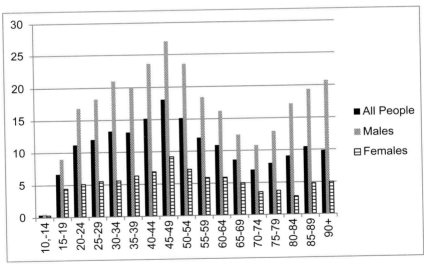

*Using the National ONS definition of suicide.
Source: Office for National Statistics, Suicides in the UK: 2018 registrations: Registered deaths in the UK from suicide analysed by sex, age, area of usual residence of the deceased and suicide method, published 2019.

Fig. 4. Number of People Receiving Talking Therapies in the Community Under the Improving Access to Talking Therapies (IAPT) Programme 2012 – 2019 and Recovery Rates Achieved

Year	People Receiving 'IAPT' Community Talking Therapies*	Recovery Rate**
2018 / 19	1,092,296	52.1%
2017 / 18	1,009,035	50.8%
2016 / 17	965,379	49.3%
2015 / 16	953,522	46.3%
2014 / 15	815,665	44.8%
2013 / 14	709,117	45.0%
2012 / 13	434,247	42.8%

* Uses the national definition of 'Entering Therapy' mandated for IAPT services.
** Uses the national definition of 'Moving to Recovery' mandated for IAPT services.
Source: NHS Digital and the Health and Social Care Information Centre (HSCIC), Psychological Therapies, Annual Reports on the use of IAPT services, 2018-19.

Fig. 5. Rough Sleeping in England, 2010–2018

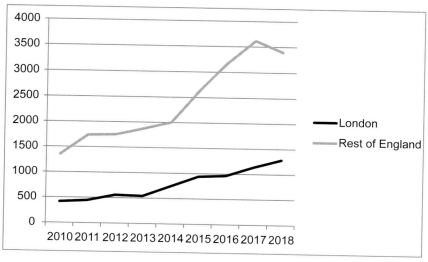

Source: Rough sleeping statistics England autumn 2018, Ministry of Housing, Communities and Local Government, as reported by the Office for National Statistics. Rough Sleeping is one component of homelessness that has risen markedly in the last decade.

Psykhe

Fig. 6. Gini Coefficient* of Income Inequality in the UK, 1979–2019

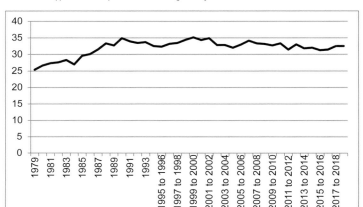

*The Gini coefficient is an internationally used measure of income inequality that ranges between 0% and 100%, where 0% indicates that income is shared equally among all households and 100% indicates one household accounting for all income. Therefore, the lower the value of the Gini coefficient the more equally income is distributed. 2019 figures shown are provisional.
Source: Office for National Statistics – Living Costs and Food Survey, Household Income Inequality UK: Financial year ending 2019 (provisional).

Fig. 7. Households with Access to the Internet*

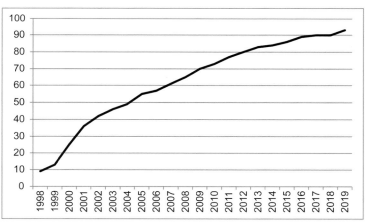

* UK collected data from 1998 to 2004, GB data from 2005 to 2019.
Source: Family Expenditure Survey 1998 to 2001, Expenditure and Food Survey 2002 to 2004, Opinions and Lifestyle Survey (formerly the Opinions/Omnibus Survey) from 2005, compiled and produced by the Office of National Statistics in 'Internet access – households and individuals', 2019.

Fig. 8. Percentage of People Using the Internet

	2012	2013	2014	2015	2016	2017	2018	2019
All adults:	80.9	83.3	85.0	86.2	87.9	88.9	89.8	90.8
Age group:								
16 – 24	97.6	98.3	98.9	98.8	99.2	99.2	99.3	99.2
25 – 34	96.7	97.7	98.3	98.6	98.9	99.1	99.2	99.4
35 – 44	94.2	95.8	96.7	97.3	98.2	98.4	98.6	98.9
45 – 54	87.8	90.2	92.3	93.6	94.9	96.2	96.8	97.5
55 – 64	77.9	81.3	84.2	86.7	88.3	90.0	91.8	93.2
65 – 74	56.2	61.1	65.5	70.6	74.1	77.5	80.2	83.2
75 +	22.9	29.1	31.9	33.0	38.7	40.5	43.6	46.8

*People using the internet within the last three months
Source: Office for National Statistics, Internet users, UK: 2019: Internet use in the UK annual estimates by age, sex, disability and geographical location.

Fig. 9. UK Social Media Usage by Age Group, 2019*

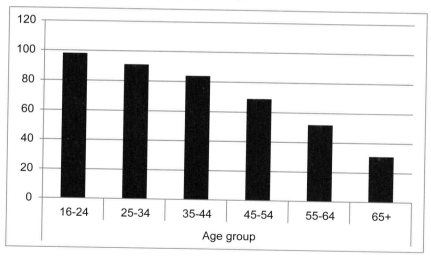

*Percentage using at least one social networking site within the last three months.
Source: Office for National Statistics, 'Internet access – households and individuals', 2019.

NOTES AND REFERENCES

The Breath of Life – A Prologue

1. Cupid and Psykhe, story from *Metamorphoses* (also called *The Golden Ass*), Lucius Apuleius Madaurensis (Platonicus), second century AD.

1 A Modern Epidemic? – A Premise

1. Revelation 6:8.
2. Estimates based on records of Roman historian Dio Cassius, see Gilliam, J. F., 'The Plague under Marcus Aurelius', The American Journal of Philology 3/82/July 1961 and Littman, R. J. and Littman, M. L., 'Galen and the Antonine Plague', The American Journal of Philology 3/94/Autumn 1973.
3. 'Plague', World Health Organisation, 2017.
4. K. D. Patterson and G. F. Pyle, 'The geography and mortality of the 1918 influenza pandemic', Bulletin of the History of Medicine, 1991.

5. Paraphrased from 'Invictus' by William Ernest Henley. Published in his 1888 book of verses. Henley's great poem was written in hospital while he was recovering from a bout of tuberculosis.

6. NHS England, 2020, World Health Organisation, World Health Report 2001.

7. Figures from the Office for National Statistics, see also Fig. 1.

8. National Institute for Health and Clinical Excellence, Common Mental Health Disorders: Evidence Update, March 201. Also NHS Digital and the Health and Social Care Information Centre (HSCIC), see Fig. 4.

9. The Institute for Health Metrics Evaluation, 'Global Burden of Disease', 2017.

10. Ecclesiastes 1:9.

2 The Emancipation of Reason – Mental Health in the Ancient World

1. Traditionally attributed to Euripides, now disputed.

2. Described by Stanley Finger in 'Origins of Neuroscience: A History of Explorations into Brain Function', Oxford University Press, 1994.

3. Huffman, C., 'Alcmaeon', The Stanford Encyclopaedia of Philosophy (Spring 2017 Edition), Edward N. Zalta (ed.).

4. 'On the Sacred Disease', credited to the Hippocratic Corpus. From the nineteenth-century English translation by Francis Adams.

5. Traditionally attributed to Aristotle, disputed.

6. Cicero, from Mental Disorders in the Classical World, edited by William V. Harris, Brill Academic Publishers, 2013.

3 *Baying at the Moon – Religion and Mental Health*

1. Genesis 1:1.
2. Edward Gibbon, The History of the Decline and Fall of the Roman Empire, Volume 1, 1776.
3. Pew Research Centre, Being Christian in Western Europe, May 2018.
4. Ibid.
5. Philippians 4:6-7.
6. Isaiah 41:10.
7. Daniel 4:33.
8. Mark 5:1.
9. Shakespeare, Macbeth, Act 4, Scene 1.
10. Brian P. Levack, The Witch-Hunt in Early Modern Europe, 3rd edition, Routledge, 2006.
11. Quote from the Vatican archive (w2.vatican.va), 28/05/2002.

4 *The Anatomy of Melancholy – An Enlightenment*

1. Robert Burton, The Anatomy of Melancholy, 1661.
2. Ibid.
3. René Descartes, Meditations on First Philosophy in which are demonstrated the existence of God and the distinction between the human soul and the body, translated by John Cottingham, Cambridge University Press, 2013.
4. 'The King's Fund Verdict: Has the government put mental health on an equal footing with physical health?' 2015.
5. '*Lasciate ogne speranza, voi ch'intrate*', usually translated as 'abandon hope all ye who enter here' is

written in Dante's Inferno as being inscribed upon the gates of hell.

6. Paraphrased from Hamlet, Act 2 Scene 2.
7. From the Diary of Samuel Pepys, edited by Richard Griffin, Third Baron Braybrooke, published 1825.
8. Ibid.
9. Wilhelm Wundt, Principles of Physiological Psychology, 1902, translated by Edward Bradford Titchener, 1904.
10. Sigmund Freud, The Interpretation of Dreams, 1900.
11. Sigmund Freud, Collected Papers V, translated by James Strachey, The International Psycho-analytical Press, 1925
12. Shorter, Edward, History of Psychiatry, John Wiley & Sons, 1997.
13. Franz Anton Mesmer, Propositions Concerning Animal Magnetism, translated in Binet, A. & Féré, C., Animal Magnetism, Appleton and Co., 1888.
14. Franz Joseph Gall, On the Functions of the Brain and of Each of Its Parts; On the Organ of the Moral Qualities and Intellectual Faculties, and the Plurality of the Cerebral Organs, translated by Winslow Lewis, Marsh, Capen & Lyon, 1835.
15. Shakespeare's Macbeth, Act 1 Scene 4.
16. 'The rest is silence' – the last words spoken by Prince Hamlet in Shakespeare's Hamlet.

5 Daggers of the Mind – Mental Health in Wartime

1. Sun Tzu, The Art of War, Section III: Attack by Stratagem, quote taken from Lionel Giles' translation of the fifth century BCE text, Luzac & Co, 1910.

2. Josef Auenbrugger, 'Inventum Novum', 1761 work quoted in The Textbook of Military Medicine – War Psychiatry, Office of the Surgeon General, United States of America, TMM Publications, 1995.
3. Bret A. Moor and Jeffrey E. Barnett (ed.), Military Psychologists' Desk Reference, Oxford University Press, 2013.
4. William D. Howells, 'Reminiscences and Autobiography', The Complete Short Stories of William Dean Howells, e-artnow, 2015.
5. Siegfried Sassoon, 'Survivors', published in Counter-Attack and Other Poems, William Heinemann, 1918.
6. Wilfred Owen, 'Dulce et Decorum est', published posthumously in 1920.
7. BBC Inside Out, 2014 http://www.bbc.co.uk/insideout/extra/series-1/shell_shocked.shtml.
8. E. F. Torrey and R. H. Yolken, 'Psychiatric Genocide: Nazi Attempts to Eradicate Schizophrenia', Schizophrenia Bulletin 36(1), 26-32, 2010.
9. Mary Soames, Clementine Churchill: The Biography of a Marriage, Mariner Books.
10. Ibid.

6 *Asylums and Agony – Institutionalisation and Experimental Treatments*

1. Ronald Kessler, 'The Sins of the Father: Joseph P. Kennedy and the Dynasty he Founded', Warner Books, 1996.
2. The Growth of the Asylum – A Parallel World, Historic England https://historicengland.org.uk/research/

inclusive-heritage/disability-history/1832-1914/the-growth-of-the-asylum/.

3. Urban Metcalf, The Interior of Bethlam Hospital, 1818.

4. A. E. Hotchmer, Papa Hemingway: A Personal Memoir, Random House, 1966.

5. Roy Porter, Madness, A Brief History, Oxford University Press, 2002.

6. Michel Foucault, History of Madness, 1961.

7. Caroline Thomas Harnsberger (ed.), Bernard Shaw: Selections of His Wit and Wisdom, Follett Publishing Company, 1965.

8. Happy Birthday NHS, Mental Health Foundation, 2013.

9. Enoch Powell, speech to the National Association for Mental Health, 1961.

10. President Donald Trump speaking in New Hampshire, 2019.

11. Mark L. Ruffalo, 'The American Mental Asylum: A Remnant of History', Psychology Today, 2018.

12. Ibid.

13. David Herzberg, Happy Pills in America – From Miltown to Prozac, Johns Hopkins University Press, 2009.

14. Dependence and withdrawal associated with some prescribed medicines – An evidence review, Public Health England, 2019.

15. Ibid.

16. 'Many People Taking Antidepressants Discover They Cannot Quit', New York Times, 2018.

17. R. D. Laing quoted in 'Studii de literatură română și comparată', by the Faculty of Philology-History at Universitatea din Timișoara, 1984.

18. R. D. Laing, Politics of Experience, Penguin Books, 1967
19. Ibid.
20. R. D. Laing, interviewed in 1982.

7 Industry and Insight – Mental Health and Globalised Capitalism

1. Jean-Jacques Rousseau, The Social Contract, 1762.
2. Dalrymple, William, The Anarchy: The Relentless Rise of the East India Company, Bloomsbury, 2019.
3. Ibid.
4. Adam Smith's metaphor for market forces, conceptualised in The Theory of Moral Sentiments, 1759.
5. From Winston Churchill's 'Finest Hour' speech, 1940.
6. Francis Fukuyama, 'End of History?', The National Interest Magazine, 1989.
7. Michaela Benzeval, Lyndal Bond, Mhairi Campbell et al., How does Money Influence Health?, The Joseph Rowntree Foundation, 2014.
8. Felipe B. Schuch, D. Vancampfort, J. Firth et al., 'Physical Activity and Incident Depression: A Meta-Analysis of Prospective Cohort Studies', The American Journal of Psychiatry, 2018.
9. Popular variant on Klemens von Metternich's (1773–1859) original: 'When Paris sneezes, Europe catches a cold.'
10. Employment in the UK: August 2019 – Estimates of employment, unemployment and economic inactivity for the UK, Office for National Statistics, 2019.
11. House price to workplace-based earnings ratio dataset, Office for National Statistics, March 2019.

12. Rough sleeping statistics England autumn 2018, Ministry of Housing, Communities and Local Government, as reported by the Office for National Statistics. See Fig. 5.

13. From Shakespeare's Macbeth – 'Life's but a walking shadow, a poor player, that struts and frets his hour upon the stage, and then is heard no more. It is a tale told by an idiot, full of sound and fury, signifying nothing'.

14. Joseph E. Stiglitz, The Price of Inequality: How Today's Divided Society Endangers Our Future, W. W. Norton & Company, 2012.

15. Thomas Babington Macaulay, Lays of Ancient Rome, 1842.

16. Office for National Statistics – Living Costs and Food Survey. See Fig. 6.

8 Worldwide Worries – Mental Health in the Digital Age

1. Harold Wilson in his speech to the Labour Party Conference, 1963.

2. Robert Burton, The Anatomy of Melancholy, 1661.

3. Family Expenditure Survey 1998 to 2001, Expenditure and Food Survey 2002 to 2004, Opinions and Lifestyle Survey (formerly the Opinions/Omnibus Survey) from 2005, compiled and produced by the Office of National Statistics (2019). See also Fig. 7.

4. Office for National Statistics. Internet access – households and individuals: 2016.

5. Office for National Statistics. Internet access – households and individuals: 2019. See also Fig. 9.

6. # Status of Mind: Social Media and Young People's Mental Health and Well-being, Royal Society for Public Health, 2017.

7. Ibid.

8. Michael Rosenfeld, 'Disintermediating your friends: How Online Dating in the United States displaces other ways of meeting', Proceedings of the National Academy of Sciences, 2019.

9. Shakespeare, Othello.

10. Mental Health of Children and Young People in England, 2017 Survey, published by NHS Digital, 2018.

11. J. Firth, J. Torous, B. Stubbs, G. Steiner, L. Smith, M. Alvarez-Jimenez, J. Gleeson, D. Vancampfort, C. J. Armitage, J. Sarris, 'The "online brain": how the Internet may be changing our cognition', World Psychiatry, 2019.

12. Friedrich Nietzsche, Beyond Good and Evil, 1886, translated by R. J. Hollingdale, Penguin Classics, 2003.

13. George Orwell, 1984, Secker & Warburg, 1949.

9 Foods for Thoughts – Holistic Health

1. From the Constitution of the World Health Organisation.

2. Global Health Risks: Mortality and burden of disease attributable to selected major risks, World Health Organisation, 2009.

3. Shakespeare, Hamlet, Act 4, Scene 5.

4. Rudyard Kipling, 'The Ballad of East and West', 1889.

5. Antony Jay and Jonathan Lynn, Yes Minister: A Question of Loyalty, BBC, 1981.

6. 'Bringing Together Physical and Mental Health: A New Frontier for Integrated Care', The King's Fund, 2016.
7. From Winston Churchill's 'Finest Hour' speech, 1940.
8. P. G. Wodehouse, Mike, 1909.
9. The Great British Bedtime Report, The Sleep Council, 2017.
10. Abraham Maslow, 'A Theory of Human Motivation', Psychological Review, 1943.
11. Ibid.
12. T. Psaltopoulou, T.N. Sergentanis, D. B. Panagiotakos, I. N. Sergentanis, R. Kosti, N. Scarmeas, 'Mediterranean diet, stroke, cognitive impairment, and depression: A meta-analysis', Annals of Neurology, 2013.
13. Felice N. Jacka, Nicolas Cherbuin, Kaarin J. Anstey, Perminder Sachdev and Peter Butterworth, 'Western diet is associated with a smaller hippocampus: a longitudinal investigation', BMC Medicine, 2015.
14. Anisha Khanna and Manoj Kumar Sharma, 'Selfie use: The implications for psychopathology expression of body dysmorphic disorder', Industrial Psychiatry Journal, 2017.
15. Living Planet Report, World Wildlife Fund, 2018.
16. Ibid.
17 Yuval Noah Harari, Sapiens: A Brief History of Humankind, Harper Collins, 2014.
18. Peter Singer, Animal Liberation: A New Ethics for Our Treatment of Animals, 1975.

10 Parity of Esteem – The Case for Public Investment, and the Policy Response

1. 'Global, regional, and national incidence, prevalence, and years lived with disability for 354 diseases and

injuries for 195 countries and territories, 1990–2017: a systematic analysis for the Global Burden of Disease Study 2017', Global Health Metrics, The Lancet, 2018.

2. Ibid.

3. Ibid.

4. S. McManus, H. Meltzer, T. S. Brugha, P. E. Bebbington, R. Jenkins, 'Adult psychiatric morbidity in England, 2007: results of a household survey', The NHS Information Centre for health and social care, 2017.

5. S. McManus, P. Bebbington, R. Jenkins, T. Brugha (eds), Mental health and well-being in England: Adult psychiatric morbidity survey 2014, NHS digital, 2016.

6. Suicides in the UK: 2018 registrations – Registered deaths in the UK from suicide analysed by sex, age, area of usual residence of the deceased and suicide method. Office for National Statistics, 2019.

7. 'Working days lost in Great Britain', Health and Safety Executive report of Office for National Statistics Labour Force Survey Data, 2019.

8. The Five Year Forward View for Mental Health – A report from the independent Mental Health Taskforce to the NHS in England, 2016.

9. Ibid.

10. Policing and mental health: Picking up the pieces, Her Majesty's Inspectorate of Constabulary and Fire & Rescue Services, 2018.

11. Ibid.

12. IAPT three-year report: the first million patients, Department of Health, 2012.

13. Ibid. See also Fig 4.

14. Ibid.
15. Ibid.
16. Mental Health of Children and Young People in England, 2017, NHS Digital, 2018.
17. R. Kessler, P. Berglund, O. Demler, R. Jin, K. Merikangas and E. Walters, 'Lifetime prevalence and age of-onset distributions of DSM-IV disorders in the National Comorbidity Survey Replication', Archives of General Psychiatry, 62^6, 593–602, quoted in the NHS Long Term Plan, 2019.
18. Suicides in the UK: 2018 registrations – Registered deaths in the UK from suicide analysed by sex, age, area of usual residence of the deceased and suicide method, Office for National Statistics, 2019. See also Figs 1 and Fig 3.
19. 'Silent Catastrophe' – Responding to the Danger Signs of Children and Young People's Mental Health Services in Trouble. A Report from the Association of Child Psychotherapists on a Survey and Case Studies about NHS Child and Adolescent Mental Health Services, 2018.
20. Denis Campbell, 'Hundreds of mental health beds needed to end 'shameful' out-of-area care', The Guardian, 2019.
21. Fred Osher, 'We Need Better Funding for Mental Health Services', New York Times, 2016
22. Suicides in the UK: 2018 registrations – Registered deaths in the UK from suicide analysed by sex, age, area of usual residence of the deceased and suicide method, Office for National Statistics, 2019. See also Fig. 3.
23. Ibid.

11. *O Brave New World! – A Future*

1. Alfred Lord Tennyson, 'Locksley Hall', 1842.
2. 'A lie gets halfway around the world before truth puts on its boots', often attributed to Mark Twain (disputed), also to C. H. Spurgeon.
3. Shakespeare, The Tempest, 1611.
4. New Zealand's well-being budget, described by Jacinda Ardern, Davos 2019.
5. Castlebeck, a private company, closed after BBC Panorama investigation into allegations of abuse and neglect at its care homes.

Hope – An Epilogue

1. The Population of Eyam 1664-1667, an undated publication of the Eyam Museum https://www.eyam-museum.org.uk/.

BIBLIOGRAPHY

General History of Mental Health

Alexander, Franz G., and Sheldon T. Selesnick. The History of Psychiatry: An Evaluation of Psychiatric Thought and Practice from Prehistoric Times to the Present (New York City, Harper and Row, Publishers, 1966).

Butcher, James N., Mineka, Susan, and Jill M. Hooley. Abnormal Psychology (ed. Susan Hartman), 13th ed. (Boston, Pearson Education Inc, 2007).

Goshen, Charles E. Documentary History of Psychiatry: A Source book on Historical Principles. (London, Vision, 1967).

Graziano, Michael S. A. Rethinking Consciousness: A Scientific Theory of Subjective Experience (New York, W. W. Norton & Company, 2019).

Hunter, Richard and Ida Macalpine, Three Hundred Years of Psychiatry: 1535–1860 (Oxford University Press, 1963).

Porter, R. Madness: A Brief History (Oxford, New York, Oxford University Press, 2002).

Rosen, George. Madness in Society: Chapters in the Historical Sociology of Mental Illness (Chicago, The University of Chicago Press, 1968).

Rosling, Hans, Rosling Rönnlund, Anna and Ola Rosling. Factfulness: Ten Reasons We're Wrong About the World – and Why Things Are Better Than You Think (New York, Flatiron Books, 2018).

Shorter, Edward. History of Psychiatry: From the Age of the Asylum to the Age of Prozac (New York, John Wiley and Sons, 1997).

Talbot, J. H. A Biographical History of Medicine (New York, Grune and Stratton, 1970).

Classical Mental Health

Alexander, Franz G., and Sheldon T. Selesnick. The History of Psychiatry: An Evaluation of Psychiatric Thought and Practice from Prehistoric Times to the Present (New York City, Harper and Row, Publishers, 1966).

Bakay, L. An Early History of Craniotomy (Springfield, Charles C Thomas, 1985).

Breasted, J. H. Translation of The Edwin Smith Surgical Papyrus (University of Chicago Press, 1930).

Bryan, Cyril P. The Papyrus Ebers, translation from the German (Chicago, Ares Publishers Inc, 1974).

Finger, Stanley. Origins of Neuroscience: A History of Explorations Into Brain Function (Oxford University Press, 2001).

Jackson, S. W. Melancholia and Depression: From Hippocratic Times to Modern Times (New Haven, Yale University Press, 1986).

Longrigg, James. Greek Rational Medicine: From Alcmaeon to the Alexandrians (London: New York, Routledge, 1993).

Padel, Ruth. In and Out of the Mind: Greek Images of the Tragic Self (Princeton University Press, 1992).

Spencer, A. J. Death in Ancient Egypt (New York, Penguin Books, 1982).

Religion and Mental Health

Bettenson, Henry S. Documents of the Christian Church (Oxford University Press, 1967 Edition).

Doob, P. E. R. Nebuchadnezzar's Children: Conventions of Madness in Middle English Literature. (Yale University Press. 1974).

Houston, R. A. 'Clergy and the Care of the Insane in Eighteenth-Century Britain', Church History 73.1 (March 2004).

Levack, Brian P. The Witch-Hunt in Early Modern Europe (London, Routledge, 2006).

MacCulloch, Diarmaid. A History of Christianity: The First Three Thousand Years (London, Allen Lane, 2009).

Noll, Mark. A. Turning Points: Decisive Moments in the History of Christianity (Michigan, Baker Publishing Group, 2012).

The Enlightenment and Mental Health

Andrews, Jonathan, Briggs, Asa, Porter, Roy, Tucker, Penny and Kier Waddington. The History of Bethlem (London, New York, Routledge, 1997).

Bartlett, P. and D. Wright. Outside the Walls of the Asylum: The History of Care in the Community 1750-2000 (London, Athlone Press, 1999).

Breger, Louis. Freud: Darkness in the Midst of Vision (New York, John Wiley & Sons, 2000).

Burton, Robert. The Anatomy of Melancholy (Utah State University Department of Special Collections and Archives, 1628, COLL V, Book 417).

Carter, R. B. Descartes' Medical Philosophy: The Organic Solution to the Mind Body Problem (Baltimore, Johns Hopkins University Press, 1983).

Cocks, Geoffrey. Psychiatry in the Third Reich: The Goring Institute (Oxford University Press, 1985).

Descartes, Rene. De Homine Figuris et latinitate donatus a Florentio Schuyl (Leyden, Franciscum Moyardum and Petrum Leffen, 1662).

Descartes, Rene. Passions Animae (Amsterdam, L. Elzevir, 1650).

Eigen, Joel Peter. Witnessing Insanity: Madness and Mad-Doctors in the English Court (Yale University Press, 1995).

Evans, Bergen. The Psychiatry of Robert Burton (New York, Octagon Books, 1972).

Gay, Peter. Freud: A Life for Our Time (London, J. M. Dent & Sons Ltd, 1988).

Heyd, Michael. Be Sober and Reasonable, the Critique of Enthusiasm in the Seventeenth and Early Eighteenth Centuries (New York, E. J. Brill, 1995).

Ingram, Allan. The Madhouse of Language: Writing and Reading Madness in the Eighteenth Century (London, Routledge 1991).

Kinsmann, Robert S. Folly, 'Melancholy and Madness: A Study in Shifting Styles of Medical Analysis and Treatment, 1450-1675', in R. S Kinsmann (ed.). The Darker Vision of the Renaissance: Beyond the Fields of Reason (University of California Press, 1974).

Masson, Jeffrey Moussaieff. The Assault on Truth: Freud's Suppression of the Seduction Theory (Farrar, Strauss & Giroud, 1983).

Porter, Roy. Madness: A Brief History (Oxford, Oxford University Press, 2002).

Redfield Jamison, Kay. Touched with Fire: Manic Depressive Illness and the Artistic Temperament (New York, Free Press, 1993).

Schwartz, Joseph. Cassandra's Daughter: A History of Psychoanalysis in Europe and America (London, Allen Lane/Penguin Press, 1999).

Scull, Andrew. The Most Solitary of Afflictions: Madness and Society in Britain, 1700-1900 (Yale University Press, 1993).

Shorter, Edward. History of Psychiatry: From the Age of the Asylum to the Age of Prozac (New York, John Wiley and Sons, 1997).

Warfare and Mental Health

Ames, Roger (trans.), Sun Tzu. The Art of War (New York, Random House Publishing Group, 1993).

Churchill, Winston. The Second World War (Boston, Houghton Mifflin, 1948–1953).

Gilbert, Martin. Churchill: The Power of Words (London, Bantam Press/Transworld Publishers, 2012).

Grogan, Suzie. Shell Shocked Britain: The First World War's Legacy for Britain's Mental Health (Pen & Sword Books Ltd, 2014).

Keegan, John. A History of Warfare (New York, Random House, 1993).

Shepherd, Ben. A War of Nerves: Soldiers and Psychiatrists 1914–1944 (London, Jonathan Cape, 2001).

Stafford, David. Oblivion or Glory: 1921 and the Making of Winston Churchill (Yale University Press, 2019).

Wyndham, Max, 2nd Baron Egremont. Some Desperate Glory: The First World War the Poets Knew (New York, Farrar, Straus and Giroux, 2014).

Asylums and Treatments

Foucault, Michel, J. Murphy and J. Khalfa (trans). History of Madness (London, New York, Routledge, 2006).

Healy, David. The Antidepressant Era (Harvard University Press, 1997).

Hotchner, A. E. Papa Hemingway: A Personal Memoir (New York, Random House, 1966).

Kramer, Peter D. Listening to Prozac (London, Fourth Estate, 1994).

Laing, R. D. Politics of Experience (New York, Pantheon Books, 1967).

McDonald, Michael. Mystical Bedlam: Madness, Anxiety and Healing in Seventeenth Century England (New York, Cambridge University Press, 1981).

Porter, Roy. Madness: A Brief History (Oxford, New York, Oxford University Press, 2002).

Shorter, Edward. History of Psychiatry: From the Age of the Asylum to the Age of Prozac (New York, John Wiley and Sons, 1997).

Valenstein, Elliot S. Great and Desperate Cures: The Rise and Decline of Psychosurgery and Other Radical Treatments for Mental Illness (New York, Basic Books, 1986).

Wear, Andrew, French, Roger and Iain Lonie. The Medical Renaissance of the Sixteenth Century (Cambridge University Press, 1985).

Industrialisation, Globalisation, Neoliberal Capitalism and Mental Health

Bertram, Christopher. Rousseau and the Social Contract (London, Routledge, 2003).

Dalrymple, William. The Anarchy: The Relentless Rise of the East India Company (London, Bloomsbury, 2019).

Friedman, Milton. Capitalism and Freedom (University of Chicago Press, 1962).

Fukuyama, Francis. The End of History and the Last Man (New York, Free Press, 1992).

Hobbes, Thomas and Ian Shapiro (ed.). Leviathan: Or the Matter, Forme, and Power of a Common-Wealth Ecclesiasticall and Civill (Yale University Press, 2010).

Keynes, John Maynard. The General Theory of Employment, Interest and Money. (London, Palgrave Macmillan, 1936).

Smith, Adam. An Inquiry into the Nature and Causes of Wealth of Nations (The Wealth of Nations) (London, W. Strahan and T. Cadell, 1776).

Stiglitz, Joseph E. The Price of Inequality: How Today's Divided Society Endangers Our Future (New York, W. W. Norton & Company, 2012).

Digital Health

Graziano, Michael S. A. Rethinking Consciousness: A Scientific Theory of Subjective Experience (New York, W. W. Norton & Company, 2019).

Green, H., McGinnity, A., Meltzer, H. et al. Mental health of children and young people in Great Britain (Hampshire, Palgrave Macmillan, 2005).

Haig, Matt. Notes on a Nervous Planet (Edinburgh, Canongate Books Ltd, 2019).

Status of Mind: Social media and young people's mental health and well-being (Royal Society for Public Health and the Young Health Movement, 2017).

Swart, Joan and Michael Arntfield. Social Media and Mental Health: Depression, Predators and Personality Disorders (Cognella Academic Publishing, 2017).

Holistic Health

Andrew Solomon. The Noon-day Demon: An Atlas of Depression (London, Chatto and Windus, 2001).

Naylor, C., Preety, D., Shilpa, R., Honeyman, M., Thompson, J. and H. Gilburt. Bringing Together Physical and Mental Health: A New Frontier for Integrated Care (The King's Fund, 2016).

Harari, Yuval Noah. Sapiens: A Brief History of Humankind (Harper Collins, 2014).

Jacka, Felice. Brain Changer: The Good Mental Health Diet (Pan Macmillan Australia, 2019).

National Sleep Foundation, Teens and Sleep (2017).

NHS Choices, Do iPads and Electric Lights Disturb Sleep? (2013).

Singer, Peter. Animal Liberation: A New Ethics for Our Treatment of Animals (Harper Collins, 1975).

The Mental Health Foundation, Lifetime impacts: Childhood and adolescent mental health – understanding the lifetime impacts (2004).

Modern Mental Health and Public Policy

Addicott, R. Commissioning and Contracting for Integrated Care (London, The King's Fund, 2014).

Alderwick, H., Ham, C. and D. Buck. Population Health Systems: Going beyond integrated care (London, The King's Fund, 2015).

Barnett, K., Mercer, S. W., Norbury, M., Watt, G., Wyke, S. and B. Guthrie. 'Epidemiology of multimorbidity and implications for health care, research, and medical education: a cross-sectional study', The Lancet, vol. 380, no. 9836 (2012).

Keyes, C. L. M., Dhingra, S. S. and E. J. Simoes. 'Change in level of positive mental health as a predictor of future risk of mental illness', American Journal of Public Health, vol. 100, no. 12 (2010).

Kutchins, H. and S. A. Kirk. Making Us Crazy: The Psychiatric Bible and the Creation of Mental Disorders (New York, Free Press, 1997).

Mayer-Schönberger, V. and K. Cukier. Big Data: A revolution that will transform how we live, work and think (New York, Houghton Mifflin Harcourt, 2013).

INDEX